Praise for

BE HEALTHY~STAY BALANCED
21 Simple Choices to Create More Joy & Less Stress

"If you simply want to enrich your experience of living, making your life a great adventure and celebration, then Susan's esteemed book, *Be Healthy~Stay Balanced*, was written just for you."

— SHERA RAISEN, M.D.
RAISEN INTEGRATIVE MEDICINE, SANTA MONICA

"*Be Healthy~Stay Balanced* is a fantastic resource to support your quest for superior health and happiness. Susan's vast knowledge of holistic living will motivate you to create a new, better you. Go for it!"

— JOEL FUHRMAN, M.D.
AUTHOR OF *Eat to Live*

"*Be Healthy~Stay Balanced* is a blessing! Dr. Jones has produced a comprehensive, yet easy-to-navigate guide to good health that should be read by everyone interested in staying healthy and active for years to come."

— BRIAN S. BOXER WACHLER, M.D.
DIRECTOR OF THE BOXER WACHLER VISION INSTITUTE
BEVERLY HILLS

"Regardless of where you have looked for better health and how much "dis-ease" you are experiencing now, you can begin to put it behind you by reading this book…and place yourself on a path to enjoy the life you deserve."

— VICTORIA MORAN
AUTHOR OF *Fat, Broke & Lonely No More*

"Here is a book I will be proud to recommend to all of my friends and clients. What an essential message whose time has come written by a radiant woman who 'walks her talk' and lives a faith- and love-filled, peaceful life!"

— BRIGITTE MARS
AUTHOR OF *Rawsome!*

"*Be Healthy~Stay Balanced* offers the tools you'll need to enrich every aspect of your life."

— JOHN GRAY, PH.D.
AUTHOR OF *Men are from Mars, Women are from Venus*

"If you're ready to improve your diet, reduce stress in your life, or exercise your way to vibrant health, *Be Healthy–Stay Balanced* is loaded with secrets to improve the quality of your life."

— GERALD JAMPOLSKY, M.D.
AUTHOR OF *Love is Letting Go of Fear*

"*Be Healthy~Stay Balanced* is a beautiful, clear, uplifting book. A guide to living healthfully, joyfully, passionately, and peacefully, it is also a fine example of the heart-centeredness that brings grace to life. Outstanding!"

— JOHN ROBBINS
AUTHOR OF *The Food Revolution*

"In *Be Healthy~Stay Balanced*, Susan Smith Jones provides practical, yet powerful, techniques to manage stress and help restore well-being."

– DEAN ORNISH, M.D.
AUTHOR OF *Dr. Dean Ornish's Program for
Reversing Heart Disease*

"Susan's book contains information on how to achieve health and live a balanced life. I find, however, that most people aren't inspired enough to seek information. So I invite you all to wake up to life and all its potential, read *Be Healthy~Stay Balanced*, become informed, and live a healed life."

– BERNIE S. SIEGEL, M.D.
AUTHOR OF *Love, Medicine and Miracles*

Be Healthy
Stay
Balanced

Also by Susan Smith Jones, Ph.D.

A Fresh Start: Rejuvenate Your Life

Celebrate Life!

Choose to Be Healthy

Choose to Live a Balanced Life

Choose to Live Fully

Choose to Live Peacefully

EveryDay Health—Pure & Simple

Health Bliss

Make Your Life a Great Adventure

Recipes for Health Bliss

Simplify • Detoxify • Meditate

The Healing Power of NatureFoods

Vegetable Soup/The Fruit Bowl
(FOR CHILDREN; CO-AUTHORED WITH DIANNE WARREN)

Wired to Meditate

To order, please visit:
www.PagingSusan.com
www.SusanSmithJones.com
www.SusansHealthyLiving.com
or call **1-800-843-5743.**

Be Healthy *Stay* Balanced

21 SIMPLE CHOICES
TO CREATE MORE JOY
& LESS STRESS

Susan Smith Jones, PhD
Author of HEALTH BLISS and THE HEALING POWER OF NATUREFOODS

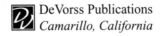
DeVorss Publications
Camarillo, California

For information, contact DeVorss & Co. at 1-800-843-5743
or visit **www.SusanSmithJones.com, wwwPagingSusan.com,**
or **www.SusansHealthyLiving.com.**

ISBN: 978-087516-836-4
FIRST PRINTING, 2008

DeVorss & Company, Publisher
P.O. Box 1389
Camarillo CA 93011-1389
www.devorss.com

Printed in the United States of America.

DISCLAIMER

This book is designed to offer information utilizing a natural way of eating and living. The information presented here shall not be interpreted or represent a claim for cure, diagnosis, treatment, or prevention of any disease. The concepts in this book have been practiced by thousands of people throughout the world as an alternative way of living and eating. The author and publisher assume no responsibility for improper application or interpretation of the information contained herein. The author believes that each of us has the inherent right and primary obligation to develop to the fullest degree our physical, emotional, mental, and spiritual potential and offers the information in this book as assistance.

Library of Congress Cataloging-in-Publication Data

Jones, Susan Smith, 1950-
  Be healthy stay balanced / 21 Simple Choices to Create More Joy & Less Stress /
by Susan Smith Jones.
       p. cm.
  Includes bibliographical references and index.
  ISBN 978-0-87516-836-4 (pbk. : alk. paper) 1. Health. 2. Stress management.
I. Title.
  RA776.J697 2008
  613—dc22
                        2008030976

CONTENTS

DEDICATION

This book is lovingly dedicated to God and to peace and the preservation of our magnificent planet Earth. And also joyfully dedicated to my two resplendent sisters, June and Jamie, and my wonderful nephews, Bryce and Tyler, who enthrall and inspire me with their loving, generous hearts and the way they all celebrate with gusto and vivacity their family, friends, and life;

...And finally to you, for reading this book and for choosing to create your very best life—to experience the highest level of health, joy, love, peace, passion, and balance possible. I salute your great adventure.

> DO NOT GO WHERE THE PATH *may lead. Go instead where there is no path and leave a trail.*
>
> — RALPH WALDO EMERSON

FOREWORD

BY JOHN WOODEN
FORMER UCLA BASKETBALL COACH AND
AUTHOR OF *They Call Me Coach*

When Susan asked me to write the foreword for *Be Healthy~Stay Balanced,* I was somewhat hesitant, but after taking advantage of the opportunity for an advance reading, I was delighted. For thirty years Susan was a fitness instructor at UCLA, motivating and inspiring students, staff, and faculty to become healthy and fit—and to celebrate life.

This book is informative and refreshing. Although Susan's exploration of "holistic" living isn't really new, she nonetheless has a special ability to take complex ideas and experiences and to present them in a clear, practical, and engaging manner. What I really appreciate about Susan is her ability to articulate feelings and describe experiences all of us have had in a way that allows us to understand our own challenges and to see more clearly who and what we are as Divine beings and how we can live our highest potential. Susan explores the elements necessary to create a life filled with positive choices and positive results. She shows us how health and happiness are not just "feeling fine" but are, as she writes, "body, mind, and spirit working as one—harmoniously." This happens, she says, as a direct result of the choices we make in life—how we eat, exercise, think, play, and rest. Yes, it is true that the choices we make in life and our ability to keep all things in proper perspective are what make us who we are.

For many years now, in my coaching, writing, and lectures, I have talked about my "Pyramid to Success," how each of us must take responsibility for our lives, and how we can all enrich the quality of life on this planet by how we choose to live. Susan conveys this message with love and a sincere desire to assist you in creating a life beyond your highest dreams. She has done an outstanding job of tying together the physical, mental, emotional, and spiritual nature of life in her unique holistic approach to successful living. She has great insight, and the world will be a better and more knowledgeable place because of her commitment to teaching the truth about health and living fully. Since I am a firm believer that love and balance are the most important essentials for a good life, I found this underlying thought very meaningful.

This is one of the most complete books I have read on how to live a balanced life. I recommend it to anyone who wants to be healthier, happier, and more at peace with themselves and who wants to make a difference in this world. I know the thousands of people all over the world who love Susan and whose lives have been enhanced by her message are eagerly looking forward to this new book. They have a treat in store. In clear and beautiful prose, Susan tells us that health and peace are a conscious choice. And reading her esteemed book, *Be Healthy~Stay Balanced,* is a vital step in making that choice.

> "BE QUICK BUT DON'T HURRY." *By that, I meant make a decision, take action; decide what you're going to do and do it. Keep this word of caution in mind: "Failure to act is often the biggest failure of all."*
>
> – COACH JOHN WOODEN

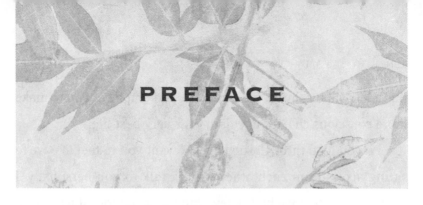

PREFACE

Life is a paradise for those who love many things with passion.
—LEO BUSCAGLIA

What a joy it is to have this opportunity to share my life and experiences on simple ways to renew your life and to create a healthy, peaceful, and balanced lifestyle. Writing a book is, undeniably, an extraordinary, sometimes difficult, yet always rewarding journey. For me, it's a process of discipline, dedication, perseverance, and commitment, and, of course, renders life-changing self-realization. Like my inviting early morning hikes in my local Santa Monica Mountains—breathtaking, bucolic, eye-opening trails winding up and down with a combination of arduous and easy maneuvers—writing a book is a similar experience, just longer. As the days, weeks, months, and years come and go, the solitary process of transmuting intuitive thoughts, ideas, research, and personal experience into a format accessible to readers fills me with ineffable joy sprinkled with intermittent heartache and immense passion. So it is with verve and enthusiasm, I share with you this book and my adventure. It is my greatest hope that my words and suggestions throughout this book will inspire, uplift, motivate, and empower you to make more conscious choices to create your very best life.

As you read through the pages, I want you to feel like we're sitting across from each other while I talk to you personally. I already know that we have a few things in common, since you've chosen to read a book on radiant health and vitality and, perhaps, to strive to be the best you can be. I am eager to share with you this program that has created success for thousands of people worldwide. It can do the same for you.

The power of choice is ours. It's up to each of us to create a meaningful, healthy life for ourselves. Sometimes that requires moving out of our comfort zone and the familiar in order to reach the acme of unbounded vitality. Yes, there is a way of eating, thinking, moving, and living, one that heals our bodies, promotes radiant health, and rejuvenates our lives.

Imagine, if you can, a life without ever feeling sick—without aches, pains, or fatigue. Imagine never getting colds or the flu or depression. Imagine waking up each day—bouncing out of bed—eager to experience life's great adventures with joy and passion. Imagine not being tempted by unhealthful foods or recreational drugs, or succumbing to noisome addictions. Imagine being your ideal weight and having people consistently praise you on how beautiful/handsome and youthful you look, and wanting to know about your diet and lifestyle. Imagine feeling hopeful, in control of your body, and genuinely grateful when you go to sleep at night. Imagine not needing to spend a penny on prescription drugs. If you can, imagine, also, feeling so vibrantly healthy that you only visit your doctor once a year or so to get an annual checkup. And imagine your doctor's surprise and delight when you show up feeling and looking younger than your previous visit. It is music to the ear to hear the doctor say that you are in superior health and have the physiology of someone twenty years your junior, and the doctor wants to learn from *you* what you're doing to be so healthy.

With knowledge and determination, willingness and courage, you can make being out-of-shape and unhealthy a thing of the past. My goal is to offer you a reader-friendly book that provides a practicable roadmap, but it's up to you to make the healthy choices. The beauty of this *Be Healthy~Stay Balanced* program is that all the things that I recommend in this book that help increase energy, boost immunity, accelerate fat loss, reshape your physique, prevent disease, and heal your body, also have the added bonus of helping to increase self-esteem and confidence, make you feel better and look younger, and bring you more peace and balance.

You may find that I suggest things that are entirely new to you, such as meditation, visualization, solitude, or spending time in nature. Maybe some of the foods and supplements, exercises, kitchen set-up suggestions, recipes, or a new way of living are different from your present lifestyle. Don't just take my word for it: check things out. Notice how you feel when you eat more raw foods—such as fresh, organic fruits and vegetables—drink more water, get more sleep, or enjoy a few quotidian minutes of peaceful solitude. You have all the answers within you. Always consult your inner guidance on every decision and choice in your life. The healthier you get, the more in-tune you will be with your innate guidance. Deep within our hearts, each of us knows the truth. But remember that active participation is important in reading this book. It's not what we read that makes a difference in our life; it's how we apply and experience the material that is of real value.

Like you, I have a myraid of things I want to accomplish in this life and I have no interest in being slowed down in any way by health issues. You owe it to yourself to choose being healthy and fit because no one is going to do it for you. You must make vibrant health on all levels—physically, mentally, emotionally, and spiritually—your top priority. Don't give up. Don't ever give up! You can do anything to which you set your mind. Move in the direction of your dreams. I believe in you and your ability to be your best, and I salute your great adventure.

> REMEMBER ALWAYS *that you not only have the right to be an individual, you also have an obligation to be one.*
>
> — ELEANOR ROOSEVELT

INTRODUCTION

Your life is really part of an unfolding plan, a charted voyage,
an exquisitely executed work of art.

— THOMAS KINKADE

Stress is a major problem in modern life. Technological advances have increased the pressure to keep busy, even during leisure hours. We talk on the telephone while we drive, watch television while we read, conduct business while we listen to the radio.

We are continually overstimulated, receiving more information from television, computers, radio, and satellites than our ancestors of several generations ago ever could have imagined! This year alone you will probably make more appointments, meet more people, and go more places than your grandparents did in their entire lives. All this manic rushing around creates a life filled with stress.

Given our current pace, we have little time to relax and cultivate relationships with our spouses, children, friends, and nature. Is it any wonder that stress-related diseases are now on the rise? Some studies even suggest that 80–90 percent of all doctor visits are for stress-related complaints. Stress-related illness is implicated in our rapidly escalating health care costs, and health problems attributed to job stress are estimated to cost U.S. businesses $150 billion every year.

I see unrelenting stress as a sickness of epidemic proportions—a "busyness" or "hurry" sickness. But you don't have to let it overwhelm you. You can choose to slow down and create a life of balance and joy. I'll address this idea in Part 2 of this book, but for now, let's see if you can find any of these signs of "hurry" sickness in your daily life.

1. Do you eat in a rush, eat while standing or walking, or eat while driving?

2. Does your busy life prevent you from spending much time at home? And when you finally get home, are you too tired to do much beyond collapse and "veg out" in front of the television?

3. Do you routinely drive too fast, run yellow lights, constantly change lanes, and jockey for position? Are you impatient with other drivers?

4. Do you talk fast, have problems communicating how you feel, and lack the time to give emotional support to your family and friends?

5. Is your life so full of undone chores and responsibilities that relaxing has become almost impossible?

6. When you're not doing something productive, do you experience anxiety and guilt?

7. Have vacations become more trouble than they're worth?

8. Do you often feel tired and run-down, cry easily, or have trouble sleeping?

9. Do you frequently get sick with colds or the flu, or find yourself experiencing one of the many prevalent diseases of Western society?

10. Do you make everyone and everything in your life more important than taking loving care of yourself?

What causes our need to rush and discount our own physical health needs? We can blame it on economics—and the need to make enough money to pay for our chosen lifestyles. We can blame it on the fact that everything's moving so fast, and we have to, too. But I believe the real cause is something deeper. By crowding our schedule with "more"—more socializing, more eating, more work, more activity, more appointments—we may be trying to fill the emptiness we feel inside ourselves.

When you constantly direct your attention and energies outward, it's easy to lose the sense of inner wonder, calmness, balance, and beauty where true happiness, joy, and peace originate. By slowing down and redirecting your energies inward, not only will you train your brain to relax, you will begin to reestablish the wholesome sense of self-worth necessary to positively change your life.

When you're under stress, your blood sugar levels can be

affected. The stress response activates the adrenal glands' release of adrenal hormones. If the stress is continuous, the adrenal glands may not be able to generate enough adrenaline to raise blood sugar when you need it. Hypoglycemia, or abnormally low blood sugar levels, may result. Irritability is one of the symptoms of hypoglycemia.

Stress often produces anxiety, defined as "a state of being uneasy, apprehensive, or worried about what may happen." According to the National Institute of Mental Health, anxiety disorders affect more than 19 million people in the United States.

How do you know when stress is getting the best of you? According to the latest edition of the *Harvard Medical School Family Health Guide*, physical symptoms of stress include headache, heart disease (two symptoms are atherosclerosis and high blood pressure), insomnia, absence of periods in women, impotence or premature ejaculation in men, digestive tract disturbances (such as ulcerative colitis, irritable bowel syndrome, gastritis, peptic and duodenal ulcers), back pain, frequent colds, shallow breathing, racing heart, herpes virus breakouts, slow wound healing, and tight neck and shoulders.

Behavioral symptoms include an increase in smoking, an increase in alcohol consumption, grinding teeth, compulsive eating, an inability to get things done, and bossiness. Emotional symptoms of stress include edginess, loneliness, nervousness, crying, and a sense of powerlessness. Cognitive symptoms include forgetfulness, inability to make decisions, trouble thinking clearly, thoughts of escape, incessant worrying, and lack of creativity.

You may not be able to change your boss's tendency to favor weekend workdays or control the bumper-to-bumper traffic to and from work, but you do have access to some powerful stress-busting tools. The simple fact that you are perusing this book tells me that you may be feeling out of balance and stressed out in one or several areas of your life. As a holistic lifestyle coach and counselor for more than thirty years, I've worked with thousands of people around the world. I offer my clients simple, yet essential, choices to bring purpose, harmony, and health back into their lives. Stress may be a fact of modern life, but you don't have to let it become your way of life. You can become the master of your life, create a lifestyle of vitality and joy, and keep noisome stress to a minimum. The path to contentment is in choosing to have your life in balance.

For easy reference, I've divided this book into four parts. In Part 1, we'll look at the physiology of stress and how it affects you. In Part 2, I'll offer you twenty-one time-tested simple stress-busters that work. In Part 3, you'll learn about the 21 "HOT" SuperFoods, and in Part 4, I offer you 40 simple, rejuvenating recipes.

EVERY BEAUTY WHICH IS SEEN *here below by personas of perception resembles more than anything else that celestial source from which we all come.*

— MICHELANGELO

I encourage you to read the book through once in its entirety and then read it a second time more slowly and see which of the tips you can adopt in your life right away. Remember, it's not what you read that makes the difference. It's what you assimilate and put into practice in your life. And it's simply a matter of choice. Choose to create your best life, and start to live with balance and joy today!

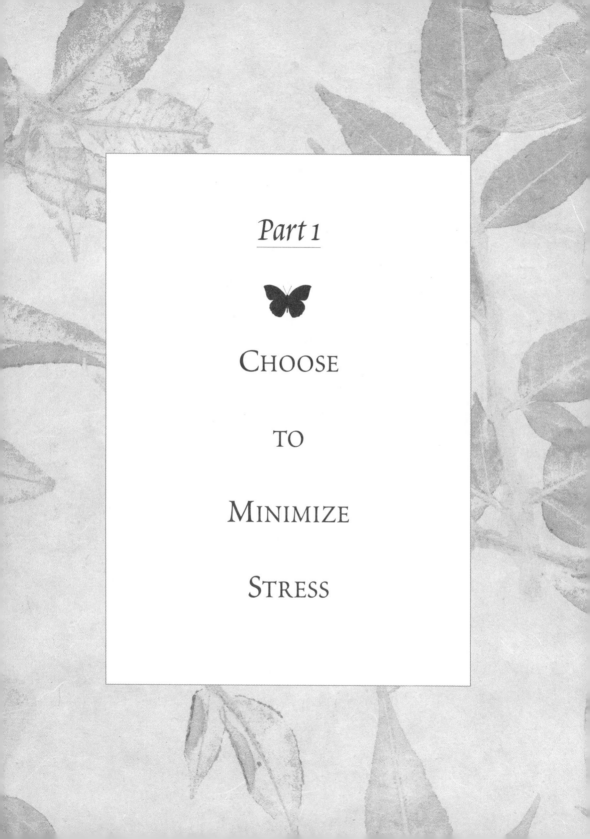

Part 1

CHOOSE

TO

MINIMIZE

STRESS

CHOOSE TO MINIMIZE STRESS

Take the complications, rules, shoulds, musts, have tos, out of your
life. This will open a channel for the genius within to emerge.
— WAYNE W. DYER, PH.D.

Not long ago, I gave a seminar in Los Angeles entitled *Be Healthy~Stay Balanced: The Power to Create your Best Life*. During my presentation I shared the essential stress-buster choices you'll be reading about in Part 2 of this book. One of the points I emphasized was the importance of putting inspiration back into your life, because when you feel inspired, you feel purposeful, and you feel empowered. I also addressed the fact that many people are experiencing a crisis of the spirit, feeling disconnected from their authentic selves—the spiritual self within each of us and its connection with Love (the Divine, God, Light, Spirit—whatever you choose to call it). I believe what we need is a revolution of the spirit, one that unfolds naturally when you begin taking loving care of yourself.

After my presentation, I went into the ladies' room and found a woman crying. I recognized her. She had been sitting in the front row of the audience and had cried through much of my talk. Since I had no plans for the evening, I asked if she would like to join me for dinner. She was surprised by my unexpected invitation, but she smiled, wiped away a tear, and nodded yes.

Melissa's story was heartbreaking. Her husband recently had left her for a much younger woman. She was almost one hundred pounds overweight, had no job, was living temporarily with her sister, and needed to find a new home for herself and her children. She was so depressed she was actually considering suicide. One morning, when she was feeling at her lowest, she took a walk and noticed a flyer for my talk in the window of a natural food store. Something inside her told her she had to attend—even though she had never attended a motivational talk before.

Melissa believed in the ideas I discussed but wasn't sure how to implement them in her life. She knew she was falling downhill, but she didn't know how to climb back up. She wanted more than anything to turn her life around—to find a job and a decent place for her children, to lose weight and get back into shape, and to live a balanced life. After listening to her story, I asked her to consider the possibility that the universe was taking everything away from her so that she could and would, for the first time in her life, put herself first. Like most women, she was so accustomed to putting everyone else's needs before her own that she took no time for herself. She was learning the hard way that you can't run on empty forever. She was being forced to learn that she had to take loving care of herself first, before she could nurture, love, and take care of others.

I told Melissa that if she were willing to make a real commitment to do whatever it took to live her highest vision, I would be happy to work with her. For the rest of that evening, I asked her to share with me her highest vision and to answer questions like: "If you couldn't fail and if you were living your best life—right now—what would that look like?" At the end of the evening, I gave her copies of all my books and audio programs and wrote out a walking and meditation/prayer program that she could start the very next morning.

Over the next month, I designed a nutrition program for Melissa that included cleaning out her refrigerator and cupboards and removing all the processed (and junk) foods that didn't align with her new vision of herself. I taught her how to shop for healthy foods and nutritional supplements, how to make fresh vegetable juices, and how to create meals that emphasized organic, raw, colorful whole foods. I also customized a cardio-weights-stretching routine for her she could do at home or at a gym. Lastly, I taught her how to visualize her goals and practice deep breathing and meditation.

Melissa's favorite stress release, in addition to taking regular infrared saunas, was aerobic dance, but she was always too tired to participate when she got home from the very strenuous part-time job she found. So we found a lunchtime class offered at a gym in an office building near where she was working. She took an aerobic dance class there 3–5 times a week. As I told Melissa, researchers found that a 60-minute aerobic dance class improved the mood of participants, particularly those who were feeling depressed (*J Sports Med Phys Fitness* 2001;41[4]). And according to the National Institutes of Health, regular exercise (even twenty minutes daily) benefits mental health by reducing stress and increasing confidence. Melissa's entire attitude about work changed for the better when she scheduled in her dance classes during her lunch break.

Melissa was an inspiration. Her dedication and commitment created miraculous results. Three weeks after getting her part-time job, she applied for and was hired for a full-time one at a florist shop. Within four months she had saved enough money to move into a large, new apartment with her very happy children.

Today, Melissa is down to her ideal weight, works out regularly, frequents natural food stores, and manages the florist shop. She now lives with a sense of freedom, control, and power over her life. She learned, firsthand, that breakthroughs and miracles occur when you are willing to live a balanced life—one that minimizes stress and maximizes joy.

A few months after he divorced her, Melissa's ex-husband said he wanted to get back together again. But she knew it wouldn't be for her highest good and said no. Soon afterwards, she met a wonderful man who supports her positive vision and they are engaged to be married. Needless to say, Melissa is feeling empowered and divinely guided.

DYING TO SUCCEED

Arthur, the president of a major American corporation, came to see me for a consultation. He also was stressed out, but for different reasons than Melissa. He was impatient, aggressive, and sometimes hostile. He was totally unaware of how to make the necessary choices to quell stress and support his well-being. He routinely put in six or seven long, pressure-packed days a week at the office or traveling on business. He always had to be first, always had to be right, and always had to be busy with work to feel worthwhile. Playful behavior did not enter into his lifestyle.

As a fancier of rich foods and a popular high-fat diet, he put away vast quantities of cheese, ice cream, steak, butter, processed foods, and cream sauces. He knew his food was loaded with cholesterol and saturated fat, but he loved it all the same. As he told me once, when it came to food he could resist anything but temptation. His exercise was shifting gears in one of his expensive sports cars.

Arthur was chronically exhausted, but he thought that if he just had more time to spend in his hot tub with a drink he could easily relax and "unwind." He had trouble sleeping at night, and experienced frequent headaches and backaches. He also developed several colds and a few bouts of the flu each year, but he assumed that was normal, and usually continued to work when sick. It wasn't until he began to sink into a deep depression that his wife urged him to have a medical checkup—his first in more than five years.

The doctor's report came as a shock to Arthur. He was only forty-five years old, but he had high blood pressure and serious hardening of the arteries (a symptom of heart disease). He was told that if he didn't make some changes in his way of life immediately, he was headed for a heart attack within six months. He also was headed toward needing quadruple-bypass heart surgery.

As providence would have it, the day after receiving the doctor's report, a friend of Arthur's told him about my holistic health private retreats and gave him several of my books and audio programs. Arthur quickly sought me out.

During the months we worked together, Arthur became a great inspiration to me, partly because his transformation was so dramatic. I had never worked with anyone quite so stressed and desperate, or who led such an unhealthful life. Fortunately, we were able to direct Arthur's innate drive to succeed toward a wholesome goal. During our first visit he made an important personal choice—he chose to make a commitment to change his life and restore the health of his younger years.

I immediately started Arthur off with meditation and mindfulness training. As I explained to him, according to studies featured in the *American Journal of Health Promotion* (July 2001), and in the cover story in *Time* magazine on "The Science of Meditation" (August 4, 2003), meditation can help people reduce the psychological and physical effects of high stress. In the study, the participants who underwent "mindfulness training" experienced an average 54 percent reduction in psychological distress after three months on the program. The group that did not receive the meditation training experienced no significant reduction in their stress. (You'll learn more about meditation in Part 2.) Arthur took to this meditation discipline like a butterfly to buddleia (that's a beautiful, colorful butterfly-attracting plant).

The other practice I prescribed for him was bodywork at least two times a week. He worked with me and a variety of bodywork practitioners, exploring massage, acupressure, shiatsu, reiki, aromatherapy, neuromuscular therapy, and energy healing so that he could determine what was of most help to him. All of these disciplines can help reduce tension, relieve headaches and backaches, improve sleep, and bring relaxation, calm, and balance back into your life. A skilled massage therapist can knead tensed muscles and help dissipate any stress you may be holding in.

Today, Arthur and his entire family are the picture of health. Recently they all participated in a 10-K run, and the following day they left on a two-week health and fitness vacation.

As Arthur and Melissa learned, choosing to live a balanced life, one filled with vibrant health, means much more than just feeling fine. It includes a quality of life, and a joy and radiance, that turns each and every moment of every day into a celebration. It's about body, mind, and spirit working as one—harmoniously. For almost all of us, being radiantly healthy is a matter of choice, because we can choose to eat and live in a way that promotes vibrant health and enlivens us on physical, emotional, mental, and spiritual levels.

It's hard to celebrate life when you're totally stressed out or when you're burdened with aches and pains, lethargy, obesity, heart disease, cancer, arthritis, and the other prevalent diseases and ailments of our society. In my decades of work as a holistic lifestyle coach, I have seen thousands of people markedly improve their health and enrich their lives through the simple lifestyle and behavior changes you'll learn about in Part 2. Before we get there, I will first provide you with a simple overview of stress and how it affects your body.

THE PHYSIOLOGY OF STRESS

Stress can be defined as a "synergy of endocrinological impairments that creates a syndrome." Loosely translated, that means that stress comes about when the sum total of your hormonal reactions to real and perceived events begins to have a significant effect on you. All day long, day after day, events in your life are triggering hormonal reactions in your body. If these reactions start to overwhelm your body's capacity to deal with them (either because there are simply too many of them and/or they are too intense), it can put a burden on you physically. Medical experts now believe that this stress-induced burden is at the root of many degenerative disease processes. In other words, stress has a biological as well as an emotional effect on you and, over time, it can diminish your body's ability to fortify, protect, regenerate, and heal itself.

Stress can affect your life in many different ways—physically, emotionally, mentally, and spiritually. Stress can precipitate high blood pressure, heart problems, fatigue, muscle and joint pain, headache, backache, anxiety, irritability, insomnia, gastrointestinal distress, and that ever-growing culprit, obesity. Although a certain amount of appropriate stress actually can be beneficial, high amounts of stress can be detrimental, making you vulnerable to illness.

Stress can be triggered by emotions such as anger, fear, worry, grief, depression, or guilt. It can be the result of a physical trauma, such as those caused by injury, accident, or surgery. Everyday pressures, like family squabbles, impossible bosses, unfaithful spouses, unruly teens, or overdue bills also cause stress. Extreme changes in your sleep pattern, diet, exercise, or even the climate in which you live can create stress. So can chronic illness, pain, allergies, and inflammation. Too much work—in fact, too much of anything—also can create stress that can lead to depression.

Stanford neuroendocrinologist and stress researcher Robert Sapolsky, the author of *Why Zebras Don't Get Ulcers*, recognizes how closely stress and depression are tied together, especially in women. Study after study has found that women suffer from both stress and depression more often than men. "Now we can begin to see how closely the two are linked. After all, depression is the archetypal stress-related illness," says Sapolsky.

Both Melissa and Arthur were good examples of the connection between stress and depression. Lisa, another one of my clients, was another classic example. Depression made it difficult for her to get up in the morning and face each day.

Lisa was a hard-working single mother of two in her late thirties, on the verge of becoming a partner in a law firm. In addition to putting in long hours at her office, she had to commute ninety minutes each way in heavy traffic. When she finally arrived home for the evening, she was greeted by screaming rap music blasting from her teenage son's room. With no time to call her own, Lisa felt like she had an endless list of things to do that never got completed.

Although she tried to watch her diet and to squeeze in two to three hours a week on her home treadmill, she was gaining weight monthly. Even more alarming, Lisa hadn't had a period in over a year. She was too young to be entering menopause, although she confessed that she felt twenty years older than her actual age.

At our first session, Lisa spoke to me through uncontrollable tears. In addition to admitting that she was having a hard time just getting out of bed in the morning, she said that she had been feeling a crippling despair for years, ever since she discovered her husband's addictions to gambling and infidelity. Just a few months after her divorce, when Lisa thought she was beginning to get her life back together, her mother died of cancer. Three weeks after the funeral, her daughter was in a serious automobile accident. Although her friends and neighbors all applauded her outward strength and ability to rise above these challenges and tragedies, inside she felt like she was losing control of herself and her life.

As I listened to Lisa's story, it became clear that she was in the midst of a severe depression. I explained to her that the physiological root of depression is often the chronic, overwhelming floods of hormones that release during times of extreme stress. I also mentioned that depresion can be viewed as a form of self-hatred as well as anger with no place to go. For Lisa, and millions of people like her, finding ways to relieve stress would make the difference between waking refreshed—and bounding out of bed ready to face the day, or waking in a fog of depression—wanting to stay in bed and hiding under a dark blanket of despair.

When you fight rush-hour traffic or face a wall of rap music at the end of a demanding day, your brain, with the best of intentions, sounds an alarm. Your heart rate accelerates, your blood sugar soars, and an army of endorphins marches out to dull potential pain. A wave of neurotransmitters—serotonin among them—spreads the alarm from cell to cell throughout your nervous system. The hypothalamus also gets in on the act, releasing a hormone called CRH that signals for the release of other hormones. Meanwhile, the adrenal glands atop the kidneys send out the stress hormones adrenaline, DHEA, and cortisol, also known as steroid hormones.

These substances are usually body-friendly and serve to protect us by increasing our alertness and strength to help us do what needs to be done. The problem comes when the stress is prolonged and the chemicals' normal routes change—serotonin tends to hasten away too quickly; DHEA can make itself scarce; cortisol can overstay its welcome.

CORTISOL'S ROLE IN STRESS & HORMONE BALANCE

Produced by the adrenal glands and commonly known as the "stress hormone," cortisol helps the body cope with all types of stress, from infection to fright, from a major job change or move to a new home, from a wedding to a divorce, and from birth to death. Whether you are facing an emergency, an accident, a confrontation, or just doing your job or getting some exercise, cortisol is there to get you up and going, to help get you through the day.

Cortisol helps determine how the proteins, carbohydrates, and fats from your diet are utilized. For example, cortisol influences the breakdown of carbohydrates into glucose so the body can use them for energy. Cortisol also influences the breakdown of protein into amino acids. Amino acids are the building blocks of protein, and they are also the building blocks of the immune system, blood vessels, muscles, and other tissues. Thus, the immune system, blood vessels, and muscles all rely on cortisol for strength and proper function. Cortisol prevents the loss of too much sodium from the body and helps maintain blood pressure as well. It also helps to suppress reactions such as pain, allergic reactions, and inflammation.

Perhaps most interesting of all, cortisol helps the body protect itself from itself. For example, during a strenuous workout, the body breaks down fat and muscle tissue to produce energy. In order to prevent the immune system from recognizing all of these tissue molecules as foreign invaders, the body produces more cortisol and gently suppresses the immune response so that the body does not go on red alert when it doesn't have to.

The cortisol that can flood your system to assist you in emergencies helps to provide your body with the nutrients you need to cope with stress. That's why it's known as the stress hormone. Typically, once you have managed the stressful circumstances, the brain shuts off the production of cortisol, your physical reactions subside, and soon you are back to normal.

But there is another side of the cortisol story. If the brain perceives that stress is ongoing or chronic, it can override the signal to shut off cortisol production. Under those circumstances, cortisol production will stay elevated as long as the brain thinks the body needs it to cope with what it is experiencing. So, as important and necessary as cortisol is, you can have too much of it. If too much cortisol stays in the body for too long, a damaging cycle can begin that can lead to blood sugar problems, fat accumulation, compromised immune function, exhaustion, bone loss, even heart disease. If, like Lisa, you experience one major stress after another—and if you haven't created ways to reduce and release that stress—it can have a detrimental effect on your health.

Just like everything in nature, the body is in a continuous state of regeneration. It is constantly building itself up, tearing itself down, and rebuilding itself all over again. Cortisol levels go up to provide the body with energy, but it breaks down tissue in order to do this. Once the job is done, the body has to rebuild and recuperate. That is when DHEA comes into play to help the body recuperate and get back to normal. DHEA and cortisol work together under normal conditions to handle stress.

Think back to the last time you felt a big rush of adrenaline. I felt it recently when I was invited to appear on a popular national television talk show. We experience these adrenaline rushes when we react to something that excites us, frightens us, surprises us, or makes us angry. An adrenaline rush is the first in a chain reaction of hormonal events. It is the signal that sets in motion the release of cortisol and DHEA, which are the hormones that help us to take action, to get a job done, and even to get our point across.

However, if you are always "under the gun"—which can mean anything from a continual struggle to make financial ends meet to traveling all the time because you are at the peak of your success in your career—then you constantly have stress hormones flooding into your bloodstream. When this happens, your adrenal glands can become overworked and exhausted. Over time, this excess wear and tear on them can be very serious, creating major disease. Given how most people live these days, it's no wonder that 80-90 percent of diseases are stress-related.

What endocrinologists have learned from studying women like Lisa, who are depressed or experiencing extended periods of stress, is that continually elevated levels of cortisol can prevent them from ovulating. The cessation of regular ovulation means that not enough estrogen and progesterone are being produced. Low estrogen levels can increase the activity of the bone-metabolizing osteoclasts. To further complicate things, the cortisol that provides the extra calcium needed in a fight-or-flight situation also stimulates the bone-metabolizing osteoclasts. Left unchecked over a long period of time, high cortisol levels can cause the body to lose bone faster than it is able to replace it. Low levels of progesterone can lead to many serious problems, including weight gain, PMS symptoms, fluid retention, depression, low energy and libido, blood sugar and mineral imbalances, and osteoporosis.

In a natural rhythm, the body produces much more cortisol in the morning than in the evening. This helps you to get up and get going, and also helps you to get through your day. At the end of the day, your cortisol level should be going down. One recent study demonstrated that when men come home from work, their cortisol levels go down. This is what is supposed to happen when you come home and wind down. However, the same study showed that the cortisol levels of women like Lisa who work outside the home and still have primary responsibility for taking care of their homes and families stay elevated in the evening. This is evidence that their bodies are responding to the stress of the "second shift." Women who have high cortisol and low DHEA levels can experience panic attacks and a strange feeling of being both anxious and exhausted at the same time.

CORTISOL, FOOD CRAVINGS & WEIGHT GAIN

Everyday pressures, recent surveys reveal, cause nine out of ten of us to look to food for comfort. In fact, almost 40 percent of Americans polled say that they always eat when they see food, and this survey didn't even factor in how this pattern is affected when we're under stress. But if you're one of those people who turn to food during stressful periods in your life, don't be hard on yourself. What at first may seem like bad eating habits, writes Pamela Peeke, M.D., a former senior scientist at the National

Institutes of Health and author of *Fight Fat After Forty,* are, in fact, "our body's natural reaction to stress. And strict dieting can actually make you more stressed out, and more prone to weight gain."

Peeke says that when you're wound up as tight as a spring, the brain sends out signals—in the form of hunger—to stockpile emergency fuel. But today, it's not because we're fleeing from tigers; it's our day-to-day stresses—struggling with overdue bills, unruly teens, inconsiderate neighbors, loud rap music, relationship challenges, illness in the family, terrorist threats, unending traffic, and other environmental stimulation. So we're left full of nervous tension, "which we often soothe by chewing," says Dr. Peeke. And that emergency fuel we stockpiled? It stays stockpiled—as fat, of course.

What's more, to create instant energy, the body drains its nutritional reserves. Under extreme stress, we need extra good quality protein (as you find in green vegetables and their fresh juices and other superior plant-based sources). What if we haven't eaten that much? The body uses its own protein-rich tissues—namely muscle. In my book, *Health Bliss,* you can read more about how important lean muscle tissue is to keeping metabolism revved, increasing fat-burning enzymes, and burning more calories, even when sleeping. And for every pound of muscle destroyed through stress, our metabolism drops, burning approximately 50 fewer calories a day.

Do you ever wonder why some people appear to thrive on stress, while others suffer ill health? New studies suggest that it may not be the stress that lowers immunity, but whether you feel a sense of control over it. In one Dutch study, scientists compared two groups of men taking a math test under a barrage of noise. Those who could adjust the noise level had little change in immune function, while those who couldn't experienced a drop in immune-cell production. In many cases, feeling in control has more to do with your attitude than your situation. And as you'll see in the tips that follow, choosing to be positive and optimistic, and reminding yourself that you're doing the best you can, will do wonders toward keeping the negative repercussions of stress at bay.

So what can we do to break the negative stress cycle? Although stress can overwhelm us at times, we can choose to take the steps necessary to keep it manageable. First, we need to understand what it means to live a balanced, joyful life. Next, we need to put that understanding into practice. Vibrant health and peace of mind (the opposite of stress) go hand in hand— you can't reach your potential for physical health without being mentally fit as well. Making choices that integrate and heal the body, mind, and spirit is what living with balance (experiencing more joy and less stress) is all about.

Part 2

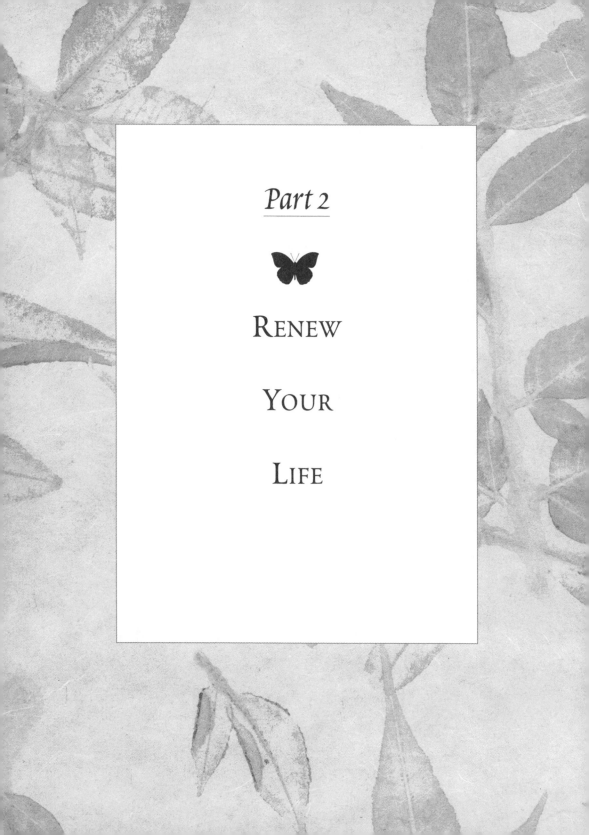

RENEW

YOUR

LIFE

21 SMALL CHANGES THAT REALLY WORK

Everyone is born a genius, but the process of living de-geniuses them.
—BUCKMINSTER FULLER

E ach of us faces tremendous challenges every day. As we get up each morning, we may face myriad stressors—getting the kids off to school, driving in bumper-to-bumper traffic, presenting a career-making (or career-breaking) report to the boss, balancing the household budget, and so much more. It can seem like there is not enough time in the day to accomplish all you need to do. These are just some of the ways everyday life can get us down. If poorly managed, these challenges can lead to many forms of stress, depression, and anxiety.

Stress is a fact of life, but you can choose not to make it a way of life for you. By incorporating most or all of the tips below, you will experience more joy and less stress. You will be well on your way to creating a healthy, happy, peaceful, fulfilling, and soul-satisfying life. Not only do these tips help assuage stress, they also help prevent and alleviate disease and depression, boost energy, and restore youthful vitality.

Living a stress-free life is not a reasonable goal. The real goal is to learn to deal with stress actively and effectively. Although that's easier for some people than others, studies suggest that anyone can learn to cope better. But I don't want you to just cope; I want you to thrive—to be vibrantly healthy, joyful, and balanced.

Here are 21 simple, yet essential, choices that I recommend and use with clients, friends, and family members to bring more vitality and purpose into your body and life. I have found them to be profoundly efficacious and practicable. Making a new life for yourself is simply a matter of choice.

So today, choose to…

1. CELEBRATE YOURSELF AND CHAMPION HIGH SELF-ESTEEM

Have you ever stopped to think about how unique, special, and marvelous you are? No one else in the world, now or in the past or in the future, is exactly like you. Never, from amongst all the seventy-six billion humans who have walked this planet since the beginning of time, has there been anyone exactly like you. As I thought about this concept recently, I thought about the approximately six billion people living on our planet. Then I figured out how long it would take to count all these people if they passed by me single file, one every second.

Imagine this. A clock ticks out the seconds while you sit in a rocking chair on your front porch. Without taking time out to stretch your legs, eat your meals, or rest your eyes, count each person passing by. How many weeks or months do you think it would take to count the world's population, one per second? You would have to sit there continuously for about 200 years! By that time you would probably be off your rocker!

This calculation of the world's population is an amazing lesson in the miraculousness of life. Try to grasp the idea that for 200 years you would never find two people exactly alike. You would never find two whose experiences had been the same or whose fingerprints were alike, or who thought, believed, felt, or talked alike.

And then to that, add the fact that you are the one special being created from one egg and one out of more than 500 million sperm that traveled an immense distance, overcame tremendous obstacles, and won a fierce and challenging competition at the moment of your conception. You are already a winner. What's more, you are composed of a body, mind, and spirit, and you already have everything you need to live up to your highest potential—to become master of your life. I think that calls for a celebration. You are amazing in who you are and what you can do with your life.

Here's an uplifting quote from Shakespeare's Hamlet that I'd like you to memorize and remind yourself of often: "What a piece of work is a man! How noble in reason! How infinite in faculty! In form, and moving, how express and admirable! In action, how like an angel! In apprehension, how like a god! The beauty of the world! The paragon of animals!"

On a universal level, I believe the thing that people wrestle with most in their own lives is low self-esteem. That's why I'm making this the first tip to consider and apply in your life. When you embrace high self-esteem and live from an empowered presence, you will be successful in all areas of your life. It's an inner change that needs to be made. Look at magazine ads, television commercials, or makeover reality shows; either by innuendo or by outright declaration, they are almost all aimed at changing who we are, making us somehow better—smarter, more attractive, slimmer, richer, and more secure. You can spend millions of dollars changing your physical features, but that will do little good until you change your attitude about yourself and cultivate a relationship with yourself that incorporates your very own divinity. When you do that, chances are you'll be happy with the physical body that God provided for you, and you will establish a salutary health and fitness program to keep your body temple in peak functioning order.

We must choose to be kind and loving toward ourselves— all the time. Self-image is crucial here. Being vibrantly healthy, living fully, and celebrating life starts with celebrating ourselves. Whether we succeed or fail, enjoy our lives or struggle, depends largely on our self-image. In fact, numerous studies have concluded that the view we have of ourselves is the key to taking control of our lives. Develop a loving relationship, a warm friendship with yourself. Be your own best friend. Out of that friendship all your other relationships form. Stop being so critical, judgmental, and unforgiving of yourself. When you are not feeling good about yourself, you feel separated from others and God. When you see yourself as a failure, you create a self-fulfilling prophecy. You attract to yourself that which you believe you deserve. Your negative thoughts and attitudes about yourself, whether they originated within yourself or others, convince you of your inability to succeed. If you feel you don't deserve success, prosperity, an enjoyable life, happy relationships, or joy and peace, you will settle for less than that to which you are entitled. When you feel unworthy, you cut yourself off from the fullness of life and create more stress. Put simply, when you learn to love yourself and take loving care of yourself, love will come to you in the forms of happiness, health, success, prosperity, peace, joy, and balance.

Living in such a fast-paced world, constantly in a tizzy over one thing or another, conspires against inner peace. The intense pace and stress of our daily lives can very easily put our peace, joy, urbanity, and health—not to mention our spiritual lives—at risk. It's easy to get caught up in the whirl of today's hectic lifestyle—especially if we've forgotten the truth of our potential. This leaves us less time for self-fulfillment. Deteriorating standards and values lead to low self-esteem and rob many of us of our dignity.

When we feel an inner emptiness, we are less inclined to make the difficult decisions of life and may be tempted to seek "easy" solutions to problems. This "quick fix" approach to life is understandable, since learning to live fully takes time and patience. But the fact is, we can, and must, slow things down if we ever hope to face our own large and small challenges with aplomb and equanimity, on terms that are our own, guided by our purest hearts. We can choose to experience aliveness and become masters of our lives, keeping in mind that this awakening is always an "inside job."

In the 1960s, Abraham Maslow wrote his famous book, *Toward a Psychology of Being,* which helped turn around the emphasis of psychology. Psychology was my undergraduate major at UCLA, and I was drawn to Maslow's work. Unlike most psychologists of his day, he chose to study high-functioning people—those living their highest potential—rather than people with problems. Maslow developed a psychology of being—not of striving, but arriving; not of trying to get someplace, but living fully. He found a common denominator among all his high-functioning subjects. They all had a vision and were committed to it, believed they had the power to master life, and were self-motivated and disciplined. Do you believe you have the power to master life? How committed, motivated, and disciplined are you to follow your highest vision and purest heart's desire?

2. EXEMPLIFY COMMITMENT AND DISCIPLINE

Breakthroughs and miracles occur when people are willing to live from their highest vision, commitment, and discipline. A commitment is the honoring of a decision. When you're committed, you allow nothing to deter you from reaching your goal. You are disciplined even when you are not feeling motivated. Making a commitment is being willing to put all of your resources on the line and taking responsibility for the outcome.

Commitment—to a project, a relationship, a health and fitness program, a spiritual practice—can lend stability to the stressful, chaotic whirlwind of everyday life. Daily actions that reaffirm commitments bring a feeling of empowerment and increase self-esteem. It's through our everyday behavior that we know what really counts. Our commitment must be woven through all of life— our thoughts, our emotions, our words, and our actions.

I know many people who say they are committed to being healthy, yet they continually let excuses get in the way. They say they'll have to wait until next Monday to exercise because they're just too busy now; they won't be able to eat nutritious food for the next two weeks because of birthdays, anniversaries, and the church's bake sale coming up; or they're too stressed to make a major change right now. Commitment means that you get past your excuses and follow through on what you said you were going to do. Make your word count. Be responsible and accountable. How do you ever expect someone to make a commitment to you or think you will follow through on a commitment to them unless you first show a commitment to yourself and what you say? Commitment takes organization, follow-through, and a big dose of mettle. If you are ready for commitment, you will be committed. In other words, you will arrange your personal circumstances so that your lifestyle, in every way, supports your commitment. You will do the things you need to do to order your life, eliminate the nonessentials and the superfluous, and consciously focus on what is important.

I know that many people wish they felt more committed, wish they had something really big to commit to. These people do not realize that you can't be committed to anything if you aren't committed to yourself. By really committing to yourself, by following through on your convictions and decisions and allowing nothing to stand in the way of your becoming the master of your life, you will quell stress, experience more balance and joy, and gain tremendous power. But to be committed, you must choose to be disciplined. Discipline is a choice. If we are to live our highest potential, we must practice self-discipline in every aspect of our lives. The mountain of soul-achievement and fulfillment cannot be scaled by anyone faint of heart or by anyone who lacks control of body, mind, and emotions.

Discipline, to me, means the ability to carry out a resolution long after the mood has left you. It also means doing what you say you're going to do.

Discipline brings freedom, joy, and balance to your life. A disciplined person is not at the whim or mercy of external circumstances but is in control of what he or she thinks, feels, says, and does. An undisciplined person is lazy, undirected, and usually unhappy. Mind discipline creates body discipline. And from a disciplined body comes an exhilarated mind.

We cannot very well discipline ourselves in the great things of life unless, and until, we have learned and accepted that discipline must begin with the small things. It's been my experience that through discipline in small things, the greater tasks that once seemed difficult become easier. For example, it takes discipline to sit at my desk each day with my water and a sanguine and ebullient attitude to write this book. As the days go by, however, the writing becomes more enjoyable, and I see my vision of a book come to fruition.

We can't address the topic of discipline without also bringing in the power of conditioning. The way we have been conditioned to behave affects all areas of our lives. For example, choosing foods that support well-being requires repeated reinforcement of such choices. When you continually repeat a negative or unhealthy habit (such as eating ice cream each night for dessert), it develops into a bad habit. To eradicate your negative conditions, to break bad habits, and to strengthen your self-discipline, make a twenty-one-day agreement with yourself. Let's say that at mealtime you want to stop eating before you feel stuffed (overeating stresses every organ and cell in the body). Resolve to stick with your agreement every day for twenty-one days. If you skip a day, you must begin the twenty-one-day cycle again. Behavioral scientists say it takes twenty-one days to form a new habit or break an old one. After twenty-one days, your mind and body stop resisting the change you're trying to make. Twenty-one days isn't a very long time. If you find your mind coming up with excuses, as it will, you can maintain discipline by reminding yourself that you have to continue for only twenty-one days.

I have been punctilious about incorporating this twenty-one-day program into my life for thirty years. On the first day of each month, I make an agreement with myself to give up some unhealthful habit or to cultivate a new or upgraded positive pattern. In this way, I make twelve beneficial changes in my life each year.

Keeping your agreements with yourself boosts your self-esteem. I know how I feel when I say I'm going to do something and I don't follow through on it. I feel lousy. When I stay disciplined and do what I say I'm going to do, I feel empowered. I have great respect for people who keep their word. I lose respect for those who don't. I have a few friends who make a habit of saying they are going to do something, like start exercising regularly or eating more fresh fruits and vegetables. But when I check with them to see how they're progressing, I hear a litany of excuses.

One thing that can undermine your ability to stay focused,

disciplined, and positive is not getting enough sleep, which leads to the next sure-fire tip.

3. SLEEP YOUR WAY TO YOUTHFUL VITALITY

There is nothing more restorative for your body than a good night's sleep, night after night after night. Consistent lack of sleep can lead to a variety of health problems, including toxic buildup, weight gain and aging, depression, irritability and impatience, low sex drive, memory loss, lethargy, relationship problems, accidents, and at least 1,500 reported "drowsy driving" fatalities each year. Studies reveal that driving on only 6 hours of sleep is like driving drunk. Cars are so cozy and comfortable these days, and cruise control doesn't help. The instant you feel drowsy at the wheel of an automobile—when your eyelids get heavy—get off the road!

People are sleeping less now than they did a century ago, thanks to electric lighting and the shift to an urban, industrialized economy, not to mention late-night television. The result is a disruption of basic body metabolism. With workloads and daily stress increasing for many of us, sleep issues loom larger than ever. Let's take a brief look at sleep and how lack of it affects us as individuals and as a society.

At the University of Chicago, Karine Spiegel and colleagues asked research participants to stay in bed just four hours per night for six nights, then twelve hours per night for the next seven nights. When subjects were sleep deprived, their blood sugars, cortisol, and sympathetic nervous system activity rose, and thyrotropin, which regulates thyroid function, fell. In other words, the results of this study show that chronic sleep deprivation forces the body into a fight-or-flight response, pushing blood sugars and other hormone-related functions out of kilter.

Higher cortisol levels, among other things, lead to memory loss, an increase in fat storage, and a decrease in muscle—the perfect combination if you want to lower metabolism and gain weight easily. But if you want to increase muscle mass, which is necessary to create a fit, lean, healthy body, you need at least 8 hours of sound sleep nightly to encourage muscle maintenance and growth and the release of the human growth hormone, which helps keep you youthful and strong. Put another way, sleeping more can make you slimmer.

Sleep deprivation also may accelerate the aging process. In the same Spiegel study, participants who only slept 4 hours per night for one week metabolized glucose 40 percent more slowly than usual, which is similar to the rate seen in elderly people. Glucose metabolism quickly returned to normal after participants got a full night's sleep every night for a week.

So how do you know if you are sleep deprived? World renowned sleep expert Dr. William C. Dement, author of *The Promise of Sleep,* says that if you become sluggish, drowsy, or fatigued, particularly after lunch or in the middle of the afternoon, you are sleep deprived. If you have difficulty getting up in the morning—one of my clients often sleeps through two alarms—you're sleep deprived.

Ninety-five percent of Americans suffer from a sleep disorder at some time in their lives, and 60 percent suffer from some persistent sleep disorder, according to Dement's research. When it comes to sleep, he says, most people require a minimum of eight hours nightly. Every hour you lose adds to your sleep indebtedness, and you cannot expect to catch up by sleeping late one day a week. The lost sleep accumulates progressively and contributes to long-term health problems. And this doesn't just pertain to adults. Children and teens actually need even more sleep than adults. Sleep loss affects how they learn, causes accidents, increases the likelihood of depression, and can lead to violent or aggressive behavior.

Recognizing that many of us simply can't get to bed any earlier or get up any later, Dement recommends napping. A few enlightened businesses are adopting the pioneering view that napping actually can promote productivity. Some companies even provide special nap rooms for employees. Naps should be recognized as a powerful tool in battling fatigue. However, if you have insomnia, naps can actually aggravate your night's sleep. By taking the edge off your sleepiness, an afternoon nap may make it even harder for you to sleep at night. In other words, if you are sleepy because of insomnia, napping should be avoided.

Naps are also not recommended after meals. It's natural to want to nap after eating because distension of the stomach from the meal increases the deep-sleep drive. The problem is that if you overeat, the digestive process may interfere with the quality of your sleep, and conversely, sleep may interfere with the digestive process. You are better off to allow digestion to occur before sleeping, since both digestion and sleep tend to work better when performed separately.

Here are five tips for better sleep.

1. Morning exercise helps you sleep at night. If you're not a morning person, exercise at least 4 hours before bedtime—any closer and you'll be too revved up.

2. Increase evening body heat for deeper sleep. A hot bath, sauna, or Jacuzzi two hours before bedtime increases melatonin as the body temperature drops. This overall increased body temperature, with its accompanying big drop back to normal, helps promote sound, deep sleep.

3. Make sure the bed is for sleep and sex only. Avoid working, eating, or watching TV in bed. Reading until you fall asleep is okay, but try to read inspirational, uplifting, or calming books.

4. Create a conducive environment. Sleep in natural fiber pajamas in a dark and quiet room, with fresh air and green plants. A cool room and cool pillow are also helpful. Two or three drops of pure essential lavender oil on your pillow promotes relaxation and calm. And, of course, a good mattress and a few pillows are essential.

5. Don't eat or drink liquids too close to bedtime. Choose your evening meals wisely. Large, spicy meals within 2–3 hours of bedtime undermine deep sleep. Alcohol is a stimulant and blocks the restful sleep experienced during the REM (rapid eye movement) cycle. While I advocate drinking several glasses of pure water throughout the day, cut off your water intake within two hours of bedtime to cut down on nighttime bathroom visits and to take extra stress off your kidneys. Sweet dreams!

4. HYDRATE YOUR BODY WITH PURE WATER

Without water, life does not exist. Before scientists look for any form of life on other planets, they first look for any sign of water. Over 70 percent of our body weight is water; that's about 10 gallons of water for a 120-pound person. We're bundles of water wrapped in skin standing on two feet.

Water is a strong solvent that carries many invisible ingredients: minerals, oxygen, nutrients, waste products, pollutants, etc. Inside the human body, blood (90 percent of which is water) circulates throughout the body distributing nutrients and oxygen, and collecting wastes and carbon dioxide. Every substance deep in our body was brought there by blood ("the river of life") and can be carried out by blood. When a person loses 20 pounds of weight through a diet program, that 20 pounds of substance comes out of the body through urine, which is why any diet program requires drinking a lot of water.

Water is very important in helping to maintain a healthy metabolic rate. At least 2 quarts a day, between meals, is essential—more if you're physically very active. That's at least 8 glasses of water daily. Freshly-squeezed fruit or vegetable juices and natural teas without caffeine can count towards your water tally. But not all liquid is alike. Some are wet but are actually antiwater. Alcohol, sodas, coffee, and other caffeinated beverages act as diuretics, thus increasing your need for more water during the day.

We often turn to food when we're really just thirsty. Water makes you feel fuller and suppresses your appetite naturally. Have a large glass of water about 15 to 20 minutes before each meal or snack. If you are interested in losing some body fat, listen up. Simply drinking purified water—between 10 and 14 glasses of water a day, and not changing anything else—not food or exercise—helps with fat loss and reshaping the body.

The liver's main functions are detoxification and regulation of metabolism. The kidneys can get rid of toxins and spare the liver if they have sufficient water. This allows the liver to metabolize more fat. Adequate water also will decrease bloating and edema caused by fluid accumulation by flushing out sodium, acidic wastes, and other toxins. A high water intake also helps relieve constipation by keeping your stools soft. Your urine should be clear, light-colored, and plentiful. Drink even more in hot weather, low humidity (such as desert environments or air traveling), high altitude, when you're ill or stressed, when you want to accelerate fat loss, or when you're pregnant.

The best water to drink, in my estimation, is purified water. A few drops of fresh lemon juice in water is my favorite way to drink it. It adds to the taste, increases the nutritional value, and assists in healing and detoxification. Lemon in hot water first thing in the morning is an excellent laxative. Make a habit of drinking water. As written in the discerning book, *Water The Ultimate Cure,* by Steve Meyerowitz (aka Sproutman), "According to a survey, the reason most people don't drink as much as they know they ought to, is lack of time or being too busy. Decide to drink purified water before every meal. Set objectives for yourself such as drinking before you leave the house, and first thing upon your return, or before you start work. Take water breaks instead of coffee breaks." He also recommends, as I do, drinking one-half ounce daily for every pound you weigh. Thus, a 150-pound person drinks 75 ounces, or approximately 2.5 quarts. Here's my general rule of thumb: Drink one glass every hour so that your urine comes out clear, not dark yellow.

5. ALKALIZE AND ENERGIZE

In his popular book, *Alkalize or Die,* author and friend Dr. Theodore A. Baroody writes about the importance of living a lifestyle that supports alkalinity. When foods are eaten, they are broken down into small nutrients and delivered to each and every cell in the body. These nutrients are burned with oxygen in a slow, controlled manner to supply the necessary energy for us to function. After oxidation, these nutrients become waste products. Gourmet or junk food, all foods make waste products. The difference between healthful food and unhealthful food is the amount and kind of wastes produced: acid or alkaline. Human cells die in about four weeks: some regenerate and some are destroyed. Dead cells are waste products. All waste products need to be discarded from the body, mostly through urine and perspiration. Most of these wastes are acidic; therefore, when we excrete them, our urine is acidic and our skin is acidic.

Most of us overwork, stay up late, get up early, and stress ourselves to the limit without giving ourselves time to rest. Most people like to eat meat and refined grains and enjoy colas and other soft drinks, which are all highly acidic foods and drinks. Furthermore, the polluted environment kills our healthy cells, thus producing more acidic wastes. This means that we cannot get rid of 100 percent of the acidic wastes that we make daily, and these leftover wastes are stored somewhere within our bodies.

Since our blood and cellular fluids must be slightly alkaline to sustain life, the body converts liquid acidic wastes into solid wastes. Solidification of liquid acid wastes is the body's defense mechanism to survive. Some of these acid wastes include cholesterol, fatty acid, uric acid, kidney stones, phosphates, sulfates, urates, and gallstones, and they accumulate in many places throughout our body.

One of the biggest problems caused by the buildup of acidic wastes is the fact that acid coagulates blood. When blood becomes thicker, it clogs up the capillaries, which is why so many adult diseases require blood thinners as part of their treatment. It is commonly known that degenerative diseases are caused by poor blood circulation. Where there is an accumulation of acidic wastes, and the local capillaries are clogged, any organ(s) in that area will not be getting an adequate blood supply, eventually leading to dysfunction of that organ(s).

Doctors have found that more than 150 degenerative diseases are associated with acidity, including cancer, diabetes, arthritis, heart disease, and gall and kidney stones. All diseases thrive in an acidic, oxygen-poor environment.

The symbol "pH" (power of hydrogen) is a measurement of how acidic or alkaline a substance is. The pH scale goes from 1–14. For example, a reading of 1 pH would be acidic, a reading of 7 pH would be neutral, and a reading of 14 pH would be alkaline.

Keep in mind that a drop in every point on the pH scale is 10 times more acid (i.e., from 7 to 6 is 10 times, from 7 to 5 is 100 times, etc.). From 7 to 2 is 100,000 times more acidic! And sodas are in the acidic range of 2 pH. Over the long term, the effects of sodas are devastating to the body. Acidity, sugars, and artificial sweeteners can shorten your life. In fact, it takes 32 glasses of alkaline water at a pH of 9 to neutralize the acid from one 12-ounce cola or soda. When you drink sodas, the body uses up reserves of its own stored alkaline buffers—mainly calcium from the bones and DNA—to raise the body's alkalinity levels, especially to maintain proper blood alkaline pH levels. Acidic blood levels can cause death!

If you want to know your current acid-alkaline balance, you can check your pH with a simple saliva test by using litmus paper that comes with a color chart. To properly check your saliva pH, bring up your saliva twice and spit it out. Bring it up a third time, but don't spit it out. Put the litmus strip under your tongue and wet it with your saliva. To find your pH level, match the color of the litmus strip to the corresponding color on the chart. Your goal is to have an alkaline (7.1–7.5) pH level. Note that it is natural for you to be more alkaline in the morning and more acidic at night.

Most of the degenerative diseases we call "old-age diseases," like memory loss, osteoporosis, arthritis, diabetes, and hypertension, are actually lifestyle diseases caused by acidosis, an overall poor diet (especially a lack of leafy green vegetables), improper digestion, and too much stress.

So how can you alkalize your body? Baroody suggests following an 80 percent/20 percent dietary rule. Choose 80 percent alkaline-forming foods and drinks and 20 percent acid-forming foods and drinks for vibrant health. His best-selling book, *Alkalize or Die,* breaks down all the foods in categories of acid, alkaline, or neutral. In a nutshell, most fruits and vegetables are alkaline and most other foods, including meat, dairy, fish, fowl, grains, seeds, and nuts are acid-forming, with a few exceptions. He recommends as an optimum diet building up to eating 75 percent fresh and raw plant-based foods and 25 percent cooked foods. He encourages the daily practice of meditation, deep breathing, exercise, deep sleep, and positive thinking—all of which increase alkalinity.

One of the quickest and best ways to improve health and increase alkalinity is to make fresh vegetable juice every day. Chlorophyll, which gives green vegetables their color, builds the blood and powerfully alkalizes the system. I'll cover the importance of juicing in an upcoming tip.

As well, on pages 253 and 264, please refer to my recommendations of Activated Air and Ionizer Plus. Both of these salubrious products will make a positive difference in your body by increasing your alkalinity, immunity, and energy, and helping to rejuvenate your body and look younger.

Another way to increase your body's alkalinity is through exposure to direct sunlight.

6. EMBRACE HEALTHY DOSES OF NATURAL SUNLIGHT

The sun is the source of light and warmth and sustains our existence. It provides the energy for plants to photosynthesize the products necessary for growth. This energy is then stored in plants in the form of carbohydrates, proteins, and fats, and is transferred to us upon consumption. In a sense, the cycle of life also can be called the cycle of light. Raw plant foods are so beneficial for us because we're taking life-giving sunlight into our bodies.

But the sun also has been getting a lot of bad press lately, and while baking in the sun is clearly not good for us, the latest research shows that short bouts of exposure without sunblock may yield significant health benefits, from helping to prevent some cancers to warding off depression, increasing fitness and libido, and lowering cholesterol, blood sugar, and blood pressure. Baroody also suggests short bouts of direct sunlight to help produce proper hormonal levels and to assist alkaline-acid balances.

Vitamin D is a fat-soluble vitamin found in limited quantities in foods; however, for most people, the best way to get optimal levels of this nutrient is through exposure to the ultraviolet (UV) rays of the sun, which triggers vitamin D synthesis in the skin. "As a fat-soluble nutrient, it can be stored in the body for use in periods of scarcity," writes Olin Idol, N.D., C.N.C., in a recent issue of the magazine *Hallelujah Acres Diet & Lifestyle*.

Idol goes on to say that for light-skinned people, "10 to 15 minutes of sun exposure at least two times per week to the face, arms, hands, or back without sunscreen is usually sufficient to provide adequate vitamin D" (*Dietary Supplement Fact Sheet: Vitamin D,* NIH Clinical Center, p. 1). Dark-skinned people require up to six times that amount of exposure to arrive at the same level of vitamin D as fair-skinned people, suggests Idol. This sunshine supplement helps prevent disease and is also needed for calcium absorption, and thus plays an important role in protecting against osteoporosis, bone fractures, and PMS. Scientific findings further indicate that because vitamin D may affect mood, lack of exposure to the sun may play a role in all types of depression, not just in the most serious seasonal-affective disorders, which tend to strike during winter months.

The sun/cancer link stems from research that found that women who live in the Northeast are 40–60 percent more likely to die from breast cancer than those who live in "sunnier" West Coast or southern areas. A new study by epidemiologist Ester John, Ph.D., at the Northern California Cancer Center, suggests that the incidence of cancer has as much to do with geography as with behavior. She found that women who lived in the South, or said that they were frequently outdoors, were 30–40 percent less likely to develop breast cancer than women who didn't fit that profile. Other research indicates that sunlight may help prevent prostate and colon cancers as well.

Experts attribute the lower risk to high levels of vitamin D, which the body produces when UVB rays penetrate the skin. Most of us don't get enough of this nutrient through diet alone. "If you live in the north, or are indoors a lot, you're at a greater risk for being vitamin D-deficient," says Susan Thys-Jacobs, M.D., director of the Osteoporosis Center at St. Luke's Roosevelt Hospital in New York.

Recent evidence reveals that sunlight also stimulates the thyroid gland to increase hormone production, which increases metabolism, which means you'll burn up more energy or calories. In the excellent book *Sunlight,* author Zane Kime, M.D., states, "There is conclusive evidence that exposure to sunlight produces a metabolic effect in the body very similar to that produced by physical training, and is definitely followed by a measurable improvement in physical fitness." He also explains in this book how a plant-based diet (vegan—no meat, dairy, or eggs) will greatly decrease the risk of skin cancer.

Just because a little bit of direct sunlight is great for your body doesn't mean that a lot is better. To allow sunburn is foolish. Immune-reacting systems are overstimulated by the action of too much sunlight, increasing body acidity. Dermatologists also prescribe caution regarding tanning beds. Nothing can match the benefits of natural sunlight. I have practiced safe sunning for over three decades. Of course, baking in the sun is still not advisable, and morning and afternoon are better times to bask in the sun, especially during the summer. If you're in the sun longer than 20 or 30 minutes, apply a sunscreen with an SPF of at least 15 or above. But for those 10 to 20 minute sessions a few times a week, expose as much of your body to the sun as possible. If you can sunbathe "au natural," do it, as you'll reap more benefits of increased vitamin D and sex hormones when more skin is exposed. Keep this in mind: If you spend just 15 minutes in the sun, you'll make approximately 10,000 IU of Vitamin D. I usually do my aerobic workout outdoors in the form of morning hiking (clothed, of course!), allowing the sun to shine on my arms and face, and, when it's warm enough, on my legs. In this way, I get a great workout in a beautiful environment and reap the benefits of the healthy, early morning sunshine.

And speaking of exercise, this is the next tip for quelling stress and living with balance and vitality.

7. EXERCISE FOR LIFE

I live in Los Angeles, the fitness capital of the world. People are so body conscious here, the first thing you might be asked when you meet someone is, "Have you got a good trainer and gym?" I wouldn't be surprised to start seeing ads in the personal columns that read: "Fit, trim, female weightlifter who bench-presses 150 pounds and has a cholesterol level of 150 looking for a tan, strong, toned man who has completed at least a dozen triathlons and has a triglyceride level of 75."

Of course, there are many reasons to stay in good shape beyond the fact that it's fashionable. Fitness is the key to enjoying life—it can unlock the energy, stamina, and positive outlook that make each day a pleasure. Along with good eating habits, adequate rest, enough sleep, and a positive attitude about yourself and life, exercise is an important facet of a total program for well-being. It is one of the common sense ways to take responsibility for your own health and life.

Develop a well-rounded fitness program that includes strength training, aerobics, and stretching. Make your program a top priority in your life, a non-negotiable activity, and stay committed to it. There is nothing that will do more good for you in terms of being vibrantly healthy, energetic, and youthful than a regular fitness program.

Never underestimate the benefits of regular aerobic exercise for cardio health. Just thirty minutes at least four times a week will help maintain a healthy weight and body-fat ratio while decreasing blood pressure, blood sugar, anxiety, depression, and insomnia. You need aerobic, or cardio, exercise to burn the fat out of your muscles. Then add strength training, or weight lifting, to build muscle which, in turn, increases metabolism. That's right, and it's that simple. Muscle burns fat. Proper exercise increases muscle, tones it, alters its chemistry, and increases its metabolic rate. More muscle means a faster metabolism because muscle uses more energy to exist than fat. Because muscle is a highly metabolic tissue, pound for pound it burns five times as many calories as most other body tissues. When you have more muscle mass, you burn more calories than someone who doesn't, even when you're both sitting still or sleeping. That's why people who build muscle have an easier time maintaining a healthy weight. They're simply more efficient calorie burners. The addition of 10 pounds of muscle to your body will burn approximately 500 extra calories per day. You would have to jog 6 miles a day, 7 days a week to burn the same number of calories. Ten extra pounds of muscle can burn a pound of fat in one week—that's 52 pounds of fat a year!

To increase muscle, you must engage in strength training, such as weight lifting or other resistance training. All it takes to add 10 pounds of muscle is a regular strength training program involving 30 to 40 minutes, two to three times a week for about five to six months. Put simply, at least twice a week or more, strength train your chest, shoulders, arms, back, and legs for at least 30 minutes each session. Then add flexibility work (gentle stretching, yoga, or Pilates™) to your cardio and weight-training routine, and you've completed the triangle of fitness. This triangle (cardio, weight training, and flexibility work) will reduce bone loss, maintain strength and muscle mass, and keep energy levels revved. Remember these three points: move, strengthen, and lengthen.

Regular physical exercise is also an effective means of reducing stress and tension. A single dose of exercise works better than tranquilizers as a muscle relaxant among persons with symptoms of anxiety and tension, without the undesirable side effects. In a classic study of tense and anxious people, Herbert de Vries, Ph.D., former director of the Exercise Physiology Laboratory at the University of Southern California, administered a 400 mg. dose of meprobamate, the main ingredient in many tranquilizers, to a group of patients. On another day, he had these same patients take a walk vigorous enough to raise their heart rates to more than 100 beats per minute. Using an EMG (electromyogram) machine to measure the patients' tension levels as shown by the amount of electrical activity in their muscles, de Vries found that after exercise the electrical activity was 20 percent less tense. By contrast, the same patients showed little difference after the dose of meprobamate.

Exercise physiologists and medical researchers are now discovering that our sense of happiness and well-being is greatly influenced by the presence of certain chemicals and hormones in the bloodstream. Vigorous exercise stimulates the production of two chemicals that are known to lift the spirit—norepinephrine and enkephalin.

A British medical team headed by Dr. Malcolm Carruthers spent four years studying the effect of norepinephrine on two hundred people. Their conclusion: "We believe that most people could ban the blues with a simple, vigorous ten-minute exercise session three times a week. Ten minutes of exercise will double the body's level of this essential neurotransmitter, and the effect is long-lasting. Norepinephrine would seem from our research to be the chemical key to happiness."

Inactivity also leads to fatigue. According to Dr. Lawrence Lamb, consultant to the President's Council on Physical Fitness and Sports, part of the reason for this has to do with the way we store adrenaline. Lamb reports, "Activity uses up adrenaline. If it isn't used, adrenaline saps energy and decreases the efficiency of the heart." The downward spiral of energy you feel at the end of the workday only will be worsened if you come home and collapse in an easy chair. "Exercise will get the metabolic machinery out of inertia," says Lamb, "and you'll be refreshed and ready to go."

Another practice that will increase metabolism, boost your energy level, help alleviate mood swings, and reduce stress on your body is to graze throughout the day.

8. EAT MORE OFTEN AND LOSE MORE WEIGHT

Three meals a day, along with two or three low-calorie, nutrient-dense snacks between meals, will control hunger, stoke metabolism, and accelerate fat loss. This is referred to as grazing. It also reduces stress in the body because fewer meals (1 or 2) with the same number of calories as 5 to 6 smaller daily meals puts extra stress on the digestive system and all of the body's cells. The results of four national surveys show that most people try to lose weight by eating 1,000 to 1,500 calories a day. However, cutting calories to under 1,200 (if you're a woman) or 1,400 (if you're a man) doesn't provide a satisfying amount of food and slows down metabolism.

The typical dieter will often skip meals, especially breakfast. This temporary fasting state sends a signal to the body that food is scarce. As a result, the stress hormones increase and the body begins "lightening the load" and shedding its muscle tissue. Decreasing muscle tissue decreases the body's need for food. By the next feeding, the pancreas is sensitized and will sharply increase blood insulin levels, which is the body's signal to make fat. And if you're insulin resistant, as many sedentary people are, you make extra amounts of this hormone (insulin) and make/deposit fat very easily, especially if you eat refined carbohydrates. Have you ever wondered how sumo wrestlers get so big? They fast and then gorge themselves with food. As you can see, this approach is absolutely counterproductive if your goal is to lose fat and reduce stress in your body.

If you want to increase your metabolism, it's best to eat several small, healthful meals each day, suggests Dean Ornish, M.D., in his salubrious book, *Eat More, Weigh Less*. This kind of grazing approach to meals keeps your metabolism stoked. It also keeps you from feeling deprived—one of the chief complaints of everyone who has ever been on a diet.

We now know that eating smaller meals more often is good

for muscle-building and weight loss. But did you know that it may even be an effective way to reduce high cholesterol? When researchers from the University of Cambridge, England, assessed data on more than 14,600 men and women ages 45–75, they found that those who ate 5–6 times daily had the lowest LDL ("bad") cholesterol levels. Those who dined only once or twice daily had the highest, on average.

For one of your snacks during the day, have some fresh vegetable juice.

9. HEAL WITH FRESH VEGETABLE JUICES

Nothing is more healing and nutritious than fresh vegetable juices. Juices are concentrated nutritional elixirs that heal and rejuvenate the body and help bring balance to all the body's cells. Juicing is also one of the easiest, most efficient, and delicious ways to ensure you're meeting your daily produce quota. Juicing is different than blending. When you juice, you separate the juice of the fruit or vegetable from the fiber. Some of you are probably thinking, "Why would I do that? Fiber is essential for good health." I agree and recommend both a high-fiber diet and fresh vegetable juices. The fiber found in raw vegetables, fresh fruits, and other plant-based foods (animal products don't have any fiber) plays a vital role in the health of the colon, the promotion of regular bowel movements, and the transport of toxins out of the body. To maximize the benefits of raw foods, we need a good balance of whole raw foods, as well as freshly extracted raw vegetable juice. To understand more clearly, here's a nutshell view of digestion.

The process of digestion begins in the mouth. Everything you eat is masticated (chewed), mixed with your salivary enzymes, and moved on to your stomach and intestines. Ultimately, the food is liquefied so that the nutrients can pass from the small intestines into the bloodstream and lymph fluid for distribution. The remaining fiber is passed into the colon for elimination after excess water and remaining minerals are absorbed. In other words, fresh juice provides pure nutrients that require little digestive effort for optimal utilization. The juicer does the digestive work in separating out the fiber, and we receive a treasure chest of nutrients in a form that's readily assimilated.

Today's commercial farming practices, topsoil erosion, and failure to let the land rest periodically mean lower nutrient density of our vegetables and fruits, suggests Olin Idol, N.D., C.N.C., in a recent issue of the magazine *Hallelujah Acres Diet & Lifestyle,* (**www.hacres.com**). Even eating the best raw fruits and vegetables may not be enough to insure an optimal level of health. In general, our bodies are malnourished, overfed, and dealing with a heavy load of internal toxicity. Our bodies are designed to be self-healing, self-renewing, and self-rejuvenating if we just give them the right ingredients, including nutrients from raw, living foods. Juicing is a simple and efficacious way to maximize our nutrient intake without putting a heavy digestive burden on the body. It also helps the body eliminate toxins.

In *The Juicing Book,* by Stephen Blauer, I found this passage by the late Bernard Jensen, Ph.D.:

> ...by adding fresh juices to a balanced food regimen, you will help accelerate and enhance the process of restoring nutrients to chemically-starved tissues. It is on these tissues that disease and illness thrive. In terms of prevention, therefore, the importance of juices cannot be overstated.

In *Live Food Juices,* H.E. Kirschner, M.D., says that if modern research is correct, the power to break down the cellular structure of raw vegetables and assimilate the precious elements they contain, even in the healthiest individual, is only fractional—not more than 35 percent, and in the less healthy, down to 1 percent. In the form of juices, he adds, these same individuals assimilate up to 92 percent of these elements.

Blauer corroborates this recommendation of fresh juices. He writes:

> Fresh juice is more than an excellent source of vitamins, minerals, enzymes, purified water, proteins, carbohydrates, and chlorophyll. Because it is in liquid

form, fresh juice supplies nutrition that is not wasted to fuel its own digestion as it is with whole fruits, vegetables, and grasses. As a result, the body can quickly and easily make maximum use of all the nutrition that fresh juice offers.

Because of the higher sugar content of fresh fruit, I generally advocate eating whole fruit and juicing vegetables (in addition to eating lots of whole vegetables). I've been an avid juicer for *thirty-five* years—my juicer of choice is the Champion—and teach juicing in my healthy food preparation classes and in workshops around the world. (See page 260 for more information or call the company at **1-866-935-8423.**) In addition to making fresh vegetable juice every day, I do an exclusive day of juice fasting once every two weeks and two to three consecutive days a month, consuming nothing but fresh vegetable juices, water, and my favorite teas. It's easy, fun, and provides the stamina I need to engage in my daily activities without necessitating much alteration of lifestyle. You just need a good juicer to take advantage of this superb health-promoting practice, and you'll read more about this in the upcoming tip on creating a healthy kitchen.

It takes a pound of carrots to make about a 10-ounce drink of carrot juice. But could you enjoy consuming that many carrots? Probably not. Yet all the enzymes, water soluble vitamins, minerals, phytonutrients, and trace elements in those carrots are extracted (assuming it is a high-quality juicing machine) and condensed into the glass of juice. The same thing applies to vegetables. You might have a hard time eating 4–7 servings of vegetables each day, but it's easy to consume the nutritional value of a variety of vegetables by juicing them.

In light of all the research on the benefits of fresh vegetable juices, it's difficult to understand why anyone would not favor the addition of fresh vegetable juices to their diet unless there is a misunderstanding about how efficiently the body handles the natural sugars in vegetable juices. Michael Donaldson, Ph.D., head of the Hallelujah Acres Foundation, conducted a study to determine the effect of carrot juice on the blood glucose levels. He found, contrary to popular thinking, that the body actually handles the raw carrot juice very efficiently, with much less impact on the blood glucose than eating whole grain bread. (You can review the study at **www.hacres.com**.) For people with blood sugar issues, adding a teaspoon of fresh flaxseed oil to the juice can further lower the glucose response to carrot juice.

Another option is to make the juice a combination of 50 percent carrot and 50 percent green leafy lettuce or other dark green vegetables. Here are just a few of the vegetables I juice: spinach, celery, beets, romaine lettuce, Swiss chard, kale, collards, cauliflower, green onions, mustard greens, broccoli and broccoli sprouts, bell peppers, cabbage, and carrots. I also sometimes add parsley, lemon, apple, tomato, garlic, and ginger. You'll find a variety of juicing recipes in my books and audio programs, which are available from my website, **www.SusanSmithJones.com**.

Keep in mind that the more colorful, natural foods you eat, the healthier and more youthful you'll become.

10. REJUVENATE WITH COLORFUL WHOLE FOODS

Of course, becoming healthy and balanced is more than merely choosing to eat wholesome, nutritious foods, but it's a good place to start. My approach to healthful eating is a diet of whole foods, as close as possible to the way Mother Nature has created them. It is this type of diet that restores harmony to the body, mind, and spirit and replenishes our life force. As Gabriel Cousens, M.D., writes in his cutting-edge books *Spiritual Nutrition* and *Conscious Eating,* "Food is a love note from God." What a glorious thought! In order to bring a sacred balance into our lives, we must choose foods that not only nourish all the cells of our body, but also feed our souls.

Our body is composed of over 70 trillion cells. Much of the fuel for our cells comes directly from the things we eat, which contain nutrients in the form of vitamins, minerals, water, carbohydrates, fats, proteins, and enzymes. Each nutrient differs in form and function, but all are vital. Nutrients are involved in every body process, from combating infection to repairing tissue to thinking. To eat is one of the most basic and powerful of human drives. Although eating has been woven into many cultural and religious practices, essentially we eat to survive.

The problem is that most of us simply do not get what we need from our modern diet. Even if you are not sick, you may not necessarily be healthy. It simply may be that you are not yet exhibiting any overt symptoms of illness. Unlike a car engine that immediately malfunctions if you put water into the gasoline tank, the human body has tremendous resilience and often camouflages the repercussions of unhealthy fuel choices.

It doesn't help that we are surrounded by bad influences when it comes to what we eat, writes Alan Goldhamer, D.C., and Douglas Lisle, Ph.D., in their fantastic book, *The Pleasure Trap*. Fast food is probably the biggest culprit. We have come to believe that any combination of heated, treated, processed, chemicalized "foods" will meet our nutritional needs so long as we take plenty of vitamin pills, heartburn medicine, headache pills, laxatives, and other remedies. "Whether you're drawn to chocolate, cookies, potato chips, cheese, or burgers and fries," writes health researcher Neal Barnard, M.D., in his groundbreaking book *Breaking the Food Seduction: The Hidden Reasons Behind Craving—and 7 Steps to End Them Naturally*, "we all have foods we can't seem to resist—foods that sabotage our best efforts. Banishing these cravings is not a question of willpower or psychology—it's a matter of biochemistry." Based on his research and that of other leading investigators at major universities, Dr. Barnard reveals the diet and lifestyle changes that can break these stubborn craving cycles—many of which are highlighted in this tip and many other of the 21 tips presented here.

Adding foods is easier than taking them away, and the simple addition to our diet of fresh fruits and vegetables will help protect the genes from being damaged. In fact, the heart of any quintessential diet is plenty of colorful, fresh produce. Driven by mounting scientific evidence, all the national health organizations, such as Dr. Barnard's PCRM (The Physician's Committee for Responsible Medicine) and National Institutes of Health (NIH) have revised their dietary advice by putting a rainbow of fruits and vegetables front and center, where they belong. Fruits and vegetables are low in calories and high in nutrients, ideal foods for healing, vitality, weight loss, and alkalizing the body. Nature has color-coded them. A simple way to assure you're getting a healthy variety of nutrients is to enjoy an attractive panoply of colorful, natural foods.

One reason for introducing more diversity of plant foods into our diets is that different foods provide different plant chemicals, known as phytochemicals. Phytochemicals ("phyto" comes from the Greek work meaning plant) are components in plant-based foods that have been proven to ward off disease and heal the body. In his superb book, *What Color Is Your Diet?* David Heber, M.D., Ph.D., head of the UCLA Center for Human Nutrition, says that most people eat far too few foods with any color in them. Studies show that the average total intake of fruits and vegetables is about three servings daily (I recommend 7–12 servings daily). If those three servings are iceberg lettuce, french fries, and a little ketchup for color, you are in big trouble. Heber writes,

> Eating is a pleasure, and we have voted with our dollars for a beige diet of french fries, burgers, and cheese. The only problem with the diet we love is that it doesn't fit our genes, which evolved over eons in a plant-based, hunter-gatherer diet with half the fat, no dairy products, no processed foods, no refined sugars, no alcohol, and no tobacco.

Here is some food for thought—valuable information to enhance your brain function and improve memory. In 2004, the results from the Harvard Nurses Study extolled the virtues of eating green vegetables. Of the 13,000 women who participated, those who consumed at least 2½ cups of romaine lettuce and spinach per week (leafy greens) and 2½ cups of brussels sprouts, cauliflower, and broccoli (cruciferous vegetables) were 1–2 years younger in brain function than those participants who eschewed these stellar foods. Your grandmother was right. If you want to be smarter, you need to eat your vegetables—especially lots of leafy greens.

The food choices you make today will determine the health you experience tomorrow. Think of food as something to nourish your body temple, to bring blessings to your life as you revel in the bounty that God provides. Just perusing the produce section of your grocery store can become a treasure hunt for you and your family. Encourage your children to go grocery shopping with you (being sure to stay only in the produce section) and then invite them to choose a different fruit or vegetable for the family to try. My best-selling nutrition book for children (co-authored with Dianne Warren), *Vegetable Soup/The Fruit Bowl,* teaches the connection between the foods they eat and how they look, think, feel, and perform. (You can order this book from my website.)

Because fresh fruits and vegetables are the foods highest in water content, and because they are the foods easiest to digest, they take stress off your digestive system and are what I refer to as "body-friendly" foods, especially if you eat them in their raw, natural, organic state. Jettison processed and refined foods—anything made with white sugar or white flour—in favor of colorful, nutrient-dense, plant-based foods. According to Joel Fuhrman, M.D., in his terrific book, *Eat to Live,*

Americans have been among the first people worldwide to have the luxury of bombarding themselves with nutrient-deficient, high-calorie food, often called empty- calorie or junk food. [Empty-calorie means food that is deficient in nutrients and fiber.] More

Americans than ever before are eating these rich, high-calorie foods while remaining inactive—a dangerous combination.

I concur. The number one health problem in this country is obesity.

In addition to selecting the most nutrient-dense foods to eat, I also encourage you to supplement your diet with fresh vegetable juices and a natural food supplement (refer to my website for suggestions) to fill in any nutritional gaps. One of my favorite whole-food supplements is *Super Organic Rainbow Salad*. This is a 100 percent certified organic "full color spectrum" superfood—in capsule form—that combines healthy and nutritious superfoods along with traditional vegetables and greens for superior nutritional support. I take this several times weekly and I always carry it with me when I travel. Perfect for those of you who just don't seem to eat enough vegetables and superfoods. Rainbow Salad provides a combination of certified organic sea vegetables, tonic mushrooms, greens, vegetables and herbs intelligently combined to create a potent phytonutrient synergy. This synergy can help rejuvenate your whole body and elevate your health to new heights. For more information or to order, please visit: **www.bernardjensen.org** or call **1-888-743-1790.**

Choosing to live a healthful lifestyle is a personal decision and something you must earn; you can't buy good health. Your health and happiness are inescapably linked. "Choose what is best; habit will soon render it agreeable and easy," opined Pythagorus more than 2,400 years ago. By eschewing disease-causing processed foods and switching over to a natural, whole foods diet—with an empahsis on colorful living (raw) foods, you will be providing nourishment for your body, mind, and spirit. What a gift to give your body and your loved ones—long life and enduring health. Without vibrant health, life loses its luster. Ralph Waldo Emerson would probably agree. He gave us this true advice: "Health is our greatest wealth."

11. LOOK YOUNGER BY THE DAY WITH RAW FOODS

Scientists and doctors are now emphasizing the importance of fresh, raw foods in our diet due to the loss of essential vitamins, enzymes, friendly bacteria, and other important microorganisms caused by unnecessary cooking. Modern scientific medicine is finally catching up with traditional wisdom and helping us prevent the diseases caused by the Standard American Diet (appropriately known as SAD).

The core philosophy of the raw food movement lies in the idea that enzymes, the catalysts needed to aid digestion and nutrient absorption, are destroyed at temperatures around 118°F. Enzymes remain intact within living foods below temperatures of 118°F (ideally 108°F). Higher temperatures destroy the enzymes, and our bodies have to work harder to digest the foods we consume. Enzyme-rich foods help provide our bodies with a more viable and efficient energy source. Raw foods rapidly digest in our stomach and begin to provide energy and nutrition at a quick rate. Consuming cooked food, either alone or before raw food, can cause a condition called leukocytosis, an increase in white blood cells. Your body may respond to cooked food as if it were a foreign bacteria or a diseased cell, which causes your immune system to waste energy on defending you. By eating only raw food or eating raw food before cooked food, you can prevent leukocytosis.

While the body also produces enzymes, some researchers believe that only a finite amount of them are available over the course of a lifetime. Raw theorists state that as the enzyme supply dwindles, the body ages more quickly, has less ability to fight disease, and essentially runs out of energy. Because raw food is in its original, natural form, it is more wholesome, assimilative, and digestible. Food eaten raw puts very little stress on the body's systems. Gabriel Cousens, M.D., a raw foodist, recommends eating more raw foods for many reasons, the least of which is for their alkalinity, their high enzyme levels, and their ability to improve circulation. He says, "Live cell analysis experimentation has shown that within ten minutes after ingesting enzymes, red blood cells become un-clumped. Something is happening in the blood after the enzymes are ingested that suggests the enzymes are effective in the blood." In other words, the live enzymes in raw foods have a healing effect on the body.

In the wonderful book *Hooked On Raw,* the author, Rhio, shares that all food, like all matter, is vibrational energy. When we consume it, the vibration of the food is transferred to us as vital life force. Therefore, the more fresh and alive the food is, the more life force we receive. Most of us can't see this life force with our naked eye, but it can be measured by Kirlian photography. This remarkable form of electrophotography captures the energy field around living things, and double-blind studies have proven that awareness of this life force strengthens and magnifies the subtle energy even more. When volunteers in scientific experiments directed their healing energy into water, and the water was then given to plants, the plants responded by growing faster, larger, and more resistant to disease! Rhio encourages us to do the same thing with our foods by focusing love energy into them as we prepare our meals. I have always loved preparing foods, but it wasn't until I read Rhio's book (and books by Gabriel Cousens, M.D.) that I consciously began to bring my connection with nature and the Divine into the kitchen with me.

I find that raw food provides a far greater range of taste than cooked food. The most popular misconception is that raw food is all one texture: crunch. People don't understand that there is a whole range of textures, such as creamy and chewy. This food can be warm or cold or just cool: the right spices add heat and excitement.

As a proponent of a raw foods diet, I've eaten mostly raw foods for years and teach courses in "Living Food Cuisine."

Participants new to this way of eating and living—it's more a lifestyle, not just a "diet"—are always astounded at how great they feel after a few days on raw foods. "We have seen tremendous positive changes in our health, as well as witnessed many health benefits in others who eat a predominantly raw food diet," write Charles, Coralanne and George Nungesser in their excellent book, *How We All Went Raw: Raw Food Recipe Book.*

> We have seen major turnarounds in cancer, heart disease, diabetes, hypoglycemia, thyroid disorders, hormone imbalance, weight problems, and many other health struggles. After seeing all these benefits, we were convinced there is something powerful to raw foods.

The changes I've seen after eating more raw foods go beyond physical to the mental, emotional, and spiritual. I experience more inner peace, joy, harmony, and clarity. My eyes become clearer and more violet-blue, extra weight falls away, my skin becomes softer, wrinkles abate, and people tell me that I look younger. I have more energy throughout the day, can eat all day long without gaining weight, and feel a deeper connection with my own Divinity and connectedness with all life. That's why I often refer to it as spiritual nutrition. All you have to do is try this for thirty days, and you'll see the difference. It's hard to put into words the feeling of balance, well-being, and personal power you experience when eating a raw-food diet. The claims of rejuvenating effects are almost universal in raw food communities.

Elisabetta Politi, head of nutrition at Duke University Diet & Fitness Center, says that any way of eating that promotes minimal food processing needs to be looked at seriously. "I think people would benefit from having more raw foods in a well-balanced diet," she says, while cautioning that an entirely raw diet would be very difficult to sustain for most of the population.

I'm the first to admit that living 100 percent raw is not an easy thing to do when you need to integrate into "normal" society. And I also don't suggest that you switch your diet from all or mostly cooked to all raw foods overnight. In my books and workshops, I recommend beginning with adding 50 percent raw food to each meal. For example, you might add a juice or a smoothie with breakfast or add in a generous portion of fresh fruit to your cereal. For lunch, include a garden salad with your sandwich and a different salad at dinner with other cooked food. For your snacks, try some fresh fruit, vegetable juice, cut-up raw vegetables, trail mix, or some raw fruit pudding or raw vegetable soup. For a varity of recipes, visit my webiste or refer to my 3-book Hay House *Healthy Eating & Living* series— *The Healing Power of* NATUREFOODS: *50 Revitalizing* SUPERFOODS *& Lifestyle Choices to Promote Vibrant Health, Health Bliss: 50 Revitalizing* NATUREFOODS *& Lifestyle Choices to Promote Vibrant*

Health and my natural-foods cookbook *Recipes for Health Bliss: Using NATUREFOODS to Rejuvenate Your Body & Life.*

As mentioned above, when eating cooked food, always start with a few bites of raw food first. Or upgrade the 50 percent raw regimen to include two days a week with raw meals as many of my clients do. Maybe on a Monday you eat only raw foods all day until dinner when you have 50 percent raw (twenty-four hours on raw). Then on Thursday incorporate 36 hours on raw— all day Thursday through Friday morning. Weekdays seem to be easier than weekends for most of my clients.

If you have no desire to eat a totally raw-food diet, I encourage you to aspire to at least 60 percent, or better yet, 75 percent raw foods. From my experience, having worked with thousands of people, it seems that this higher amount of raw food versus cooked food will make a profound difference in how you feel and look. I am not a "raw-food purist." I still enjoy cooking and going out to eat, but most of the time I consume healthful raw foods. Remember, raw doesn't necessarily mean cold. Foods may be warmed to well above body temperature and still maintain their life force. A good rule of thumb is: If you stick your finger in it, it should feel warm—not hot.

In order to create many of the foods in a raw food diet, or simply make healthful cooked meals easily without spending hours in the kitchen, it's helpful to have a few beneficial tools at your disposal.

12. CREATE A HEALTHY KITCHEN

No matter how much you enjoy meal preparation, it helps to have a little help from your friends, the kitchen gadget angels, who want nothing more than to make your life easier! You can reduce your stress immeasurably by having available a few culinary tools that add to the beauty and diversity of the food and allow you to pull together healthful meals in minutes. In addition to the items described below, you will need everyday tools, such as various-sized knives, whisks, offset and other spatulas, an assortment of sieves and colanders, a variety of mixing bowls and spoons, a salad spinner, a couple microplanes, nonstick pans, a sushi mat, a citrus reamer, food processor (large and small), a garlic press, and a quality set of cookware. But to take it to the next level, consider adding these to your healthy kitchen.

BLENDER. A high-speed blender is a must for any kitchen and at the top of the list for me because it can be used in many different capacities, such as making soups, smoothies, creams, sauces, dressings, purées, nut milks, ice cream, nut butters, and seed meal. Inexpensive blenders can make simple dressings and sauces but are unable to make creamy smoothies, chop ice, or make butters from seeds and nuts. This is one time you want to invest in the very best, which is the Total Blender™. No other blender offers the power, ease of operation, and state-of-the-art engineering. The half-gallon capacity jar is lightweight and easy to clean, and the powerful 3-peak horsepower motor makes any blending chore a breeze. I use it at home, in my healthy cuisine classes, and on television shows. This computer-controlled blender breaks down even the toughest fibers in fruits/vegetables and is incomparable for making creamy dressings, soups, sorbets, ice creams, and more. For more information, or to order, visit my website, click on *Susan's Favorite Products,* and then click on Blendtec.

CITRUS JUICER. Available in manual or electric. It's a handy gadget for extracting juice.

CUTTING BOARDS. A wooden cutting board is best. It is nontoxic and food-safe. It does absorb flavors, so it is best to wash between uses or to have separate boards for fruits and vegetables and for animal products.

DEHYDRATOR. This is a great tool for making seasoned sprouted nuts and seeds, breads and chips, fruit leathers, and dried fruits and vegetables. It will warm and dry foods at low temperatures and can be used for "cooking" foods without destroying their entire enzyme content. The best dehydrator, and the only one that I use and recommend, the Excalibur (**www.drying123.com**) has a fan and a heating element in the rear. Stackable dryers are less efficient and can under- or over-dry foods.

FOOD PROCESSOR. A wonderful time-saving aid in the kitchen. It can chop, dice, and slice large amounts of food very quickly. It is powerful enough to grind nuts and seeds into powder.

HYDRO FLOSS®. You may think it's strange to mention the Hydro Floss oral irrigator in the section about setting up a healthy kitchen. Well, in my home, this is where I use it. With recent studies revealing the link between gum disease and several life-threatening diseases, including heart disease, stroke, and diabetes, our attention to our oral health is vital. The Hydro Floss oral irrigator provides the extra cleaning ability that complements and completes brushing and flossing. This durable and user-friendly tool flushes unwanted plaque and bacteria from the mouth. After using the Hydro Floss, you feel the difference; your teeth feel alive and sparkling clean. I wouldn't be without mine, and I even take it with me when I travel. (For more information or to order, please call: **1-800-635-3594** or visit: **www.OralCareTech.com**)

JUICER. This is essential for turning delicious fruits and vegetables into juices loaded with nutrients and flavors. Don't get a centrifugal or spinning juicer, which are the most common ones available on the market. They lack efficiency and extract only about 60 percent of the juice. They also cause the juice to quickly oxidize, and the juice may require straining. Moreover, all they do is juice. You'd be better off purchasing a multi-purpose triturating or homogenizing juicer so that you also can make nut butters, nut cheeses, baby foods, ice creams, pâtés, and other delights.

For over 35 years, I've used and recommended the Champion Juicer. Created with simplicity in mind, the Champion doesn't require nuts, bolts, screws or clamps. Assembly can be completed in seconds; cleaning is equally quick and easy. This machine is designed to produce the highest quality fruit and vegetable juices and foods. It's a difference you can see in the color of the fresh juice: darker, richer colors contain more of the pigments—and it's a difference you can taste, too. For more information or to order, please refer to my website, click on *Susan's Favorite Products,* and read my article on "The Healing Power of Fresh Juices," or listen to the radio interview. You can also call the company at **1-866-935-8423.**

KNIVES. There are three knives everyone needs in their kitchen. A paring knife is a small one for peeling and exact cutting. A chopping knife is large and heavy and is used for mincing and dicing. A chef's knife is long and wide—used for slicing. With these three, you have it made, but be sure to keep them sharp.

MANDOLINE. A breeze to use if you want to slice vegetables and fruits in a number of ways—from strips to crinkle cut. I appreciate its simplicity, manual function, and quiet operation, and it also affords me an upper body workout.

SPIRALIZER. A (manual) device that enables you to transform vegetables into long strands of angel hair pasta and other beautiful designs. It's a great way to make raw pasta and other treats. (**www.livingnutrition.com/healthshop.html** or **1-707-827-3496.**)

SPICE GRINDER. I use a variety of spice grinders, from an old-fashioned mortar and pestle to an electric-powered grinder. The electric one quickly transforms the toughest seeds and grains into a fine power and is powerful enough to make pastes. It is also easier to clean than a coffee grinder.

SPROUTING JAR AND BAG. A glass jar, covered with a screen or mesh, is used to grow sprouts. A mesh bag, with a drawstring, is used for sprouting, making nut and seed cheese, straining nut or coconut milk, or for removing the fine hairs from mango nectar or ground gingerroot.

After spending time in the kitchen preparing delicious, healthy meals, you deserve some time to relax.

13. PRACTICE THE ART OF RELAXATION AND DEEP BREATHING

One of the world's leading experts on the brain is a Harvard medical doctor, Herbert Benson, M.D., author of *The Relaxation Response* and *Your Maximum Mind.* What Benson calls "the relaxation response" is the body's ability to enter into a state characterized by an overall reduction of the metabolic rate and a lowered heart rate. According to Benson, this state of relaxation also acts as a door to a renewed mind, a changed life, and a feeling of awareness. He describes the physiological changes that occur when you are relaxed as a harmonizing or increased communication between the two sides of the brain, resulting in feelings often described as well-being, unboundedness, infinite connection, and peak experience.

One way to cultivate calmness and peacefulness is to progressively relax your body, beginning with your toes and ending with your head. Breathe slowly and deeply, and totally relax each part of your body, saying to yourself as you go along, "My toes, feet, legs [and so on] are relaxed," until you have gone through your entire body. Then rest for a while in the quiet and silence. Listening to a relaxation or meditation tape also may be helpful. (You can find out more about my own relaxation tapes by visiting my website.)

Here's another great tip you can easily do at work or at home to help relax your mind and body. Look at a picture of a beautiful landscape. Yes, it's that simple! Two studies measured the effect of certain photographic images on emotional and physiological responses. The first study was designed to find ways of fighting the boredom and homesickness that astronauts experience during extended stays in space. Researchers projected a variety of slides on the walls of a room built to simulate a space station and recorded the subjects' responses to various scenes. The second study focused on hospital patients who were about to undergo surgery. In both groups, pictures of spacious views and glistening water lowered heart rates and produced feelings of calmness.

An easy and inexpensive way to look at a beautiful landscape is to get a poster. I have a Sierra Club poster in my meditation room that has a dazzling view of water, mountains, and colorful wildflowers. Every time I look at it, I feel more relaxed. This is the perfect solution if you work in an office without windows. Larger posters of resplendent nature scenes can transform a room and provide you with a mini-fantasy vacation whenever you need it.

I also highly recommend getting one of those "sound soothers" that offer a variety of nature sounds, everything from gentle rain, to ocean waves, and a flowing brook, to a waterfall, an aviary, and windchimes. I use mine daily.

Can you breathe your way to vibrant health with deep breathing exercises? In most cases, I think you can. How often do you pause to consider the intricacies of breathing? Breathing is perhaps the only physiological process that can be either voluntary or involuntary. One can breathe, making their breath do whatever they wish, or one can ignore it, and after a while the body simply begins to breathe on its own. Breathing becomes reflexive. The body can't operate without breathing, so if conscious control of the breath is abandoned, then some unconscious part of the mind begins functioning, picks it up and starts breathing for us. Something is triggered in the lower part of the brain. But in this case, breathing falls back under the control of primitive parts of the brain, the unconscious realms of the mind, where emotions, thoughts and feelings (of which we may have little or no awareness) become involved. These wreak havoc with breath rhythms. In other words, the breath becomes haphazard and often irregular if we lose conscious control of it. It's important to bring breath back into your awareness so it's re-integrated into your consciousness.

Are your breaths rapid and shallow? Take a minute now to check and see how many breaths per minute you take (count both the inhalation and exhalation as one breath). If it is between 16–20, then you are most likely a thoracic breather. This means that your breaths are not getting to the lower part of your lungs but remain fairly high in the chest. Thoracic breathing is the least efficient and most common type.

Diaphragmatic or deep abdominal breathing, on the other hand, promotes a more relaxed state. Take a long, slow, deep breath right now. Visualize the air filling the lower part of the lungs. Since gravity pulls more blood into that area, the most efficient passage of oxygen into the blood occurs there, slowing the breath as the body gets more oxygen. It's important to note how closely tied are respiration and the heart. As the breath slows (to 6–8 breaths per minute) and deepens, the heart's job is made considerably easier. There is evidence to suggest that diaphragmatic breathing is beneficial because it increases the suction pressure created in the thoracic cavity and improves the venous return of blood, thereby reducing the load on the heart and enhancing circulatory function. Also, diaphragmatic breathing has the added bonus of relaxing the muscles of the ribs, chest, and stomach.

Diaphragmatic breathing is really quite simple. It's the habit of doing it that must be consciouslly cultivated before it can become automatic. A simple practice to achieve this is to lie down on your back on your bed or a mat or rug, with one palm placed on the center of the chest and the other on the lower edge of the rib cage where the abdomnen begins. As you inhale, the lower edge of the rib cage should expand and the abdomen should rise; as you exhale, the opposite should occur; there should be relatively little movement of the upper chest. By practicing diaphragmatic breathing, you will find in time that this exercise is becoming habitual and automatic.

So choose to cultiate the habit of deep breathing. In order to make deep breathing automatic in my life, I tried this experiement several years ago. I set my watch to beep every hour (except when I was sleeping, of course) and I took one to three minutes to do some deep breathing. As the days and weeks went on, I noticed that when the hourly beep came around, I was already practicing deep breathing; it was increaingly becoming a habit. Now, most of the time, diaphragmatic breathing is my natural way to breathe.

Simply put: Developing harmonious and rhythmic breathing along with diaphragmatic breathing will have health benefits and can improve your quality of life. But even the best diaphragmatic breathing cannot stop the cellular aging process. As you age, your cells become less able to use the oxygen in the air to generate cell energy. My advice is to optimize your breathing and enhance the air you breathe with Activated Air by Eng3. This natural solution makes oxygen more available to your cells for better mental and physical performance, healthy aging, and for repairing the damage of excessive free radicals. For more information, please refer to pages 253, or visit: **www.eng3corp.com**.

I have always found that when I'm relaxed, calm and balanced and have been breathing deeply on a regular basis, it's easier to live in the moment and laugh at myself and all the incongruities of daily life.

14. BE IN THE PRECIOUS PRESENT AND LAUGH OFTEN

Living in the moment is different from living for the moment. Young children seem to be masters of getting totally involved in and focused on whatever they are doing right now. Granted, their attention span is not long, but they are able to focus on whatever is taking place in their lives at the moment. When they eat, they just eat; when they play, they just play; when they talk, they just talk. They throw themselves wholeheartedly into their activities.

Have you ever noticed that young children are willing to try anything at a moment's notice? Even though they might have experienced that same thing before, they will express wide-eyed excitement and wonderment. Children don't use a yardstick to measure activities or compare the present with the past. They know they've played the game before, or had someone read the same story just last night, yet the game or the story is still as fresh and as wonderful as it was the first time.

Think about your attitude when doing the dishes, vacuuming, or watering the plants. You probably find these activities boring. But a child can't wait to participate, and acts as though it's just about the most exciting thing he or she has ever done. What a wonderful quality that is! To be excited about life—about every part of life as though it's always fresh and new. Actually, it is. It's only old thoughts and distorted attitudes that get in the way of celebrating each moment.

One way to be mindful of the present moment is to focus on your breathing, as elucidated above. "Conscious breathing, which is a powerful meditation in its own right," writes Eckhart Tolle in the sagacious book, *The Power of Now,* will gradually put you in touch with the body. Follow the breath with your attention as it moves in and out of your body. Breathe into the body, and feel your abdomen expanding and contracting slightly with each inhalation and exhalation. If you find it easy to visualize, close your eyes and see yourself surrounded by light or immersed in a luminous substance—a sea of consciousness. Then breathe in that light.

I do this exercise a few times each day to help me remember to be in the present moment.

This precious present moment is the only moment we'll ever have. It's our moment of power and all there is in life. In this moment, problems do not exist. It is here we find our joy and balance and are able to embrace our true selves. It is here we discover that we are already complete and perfect, according to Tolle. If we are able to be fully present and take each step in the "Now," we will be opening ourselves to the transforming experience of the power of the present. "When your attention is in the present moment, you enjoy life more intensely because you are fully alive," writes Don Miguel Ruiz in another one of my favorite books, *The Four Agreements*. I like that a lot. You enjoy life more intensely because you are fully alive! How alive and present are you to the Now in your life?

Have you ever driven to work or run errands and not

remembered how you got there? Check in with yourself every hour or so. Are you slouching? How's your attitude? What are you thinking? Is your breathing shallow? Don't wait until your shoulders are up around your ears before you try to relax. Learn to be mindful about how you're feeling and what's happening around you. I usually describe mindfulness as developing the mind's capacity to attain a balanced, awake understanding of what's happening, knowing how you feel about it, and choosing your wisest response. In my estimation, your wisest response— no matter what's going on in your life at the moment—is to embrace a cheerful attitude.

Along with my faith in God, meditation/prayer time, being in nature, and living in the present moment, laughter is another one of my favorite ways to mollify stress. It is okay to laugh, even when times are tough. Toxic worry almost always entails a loss of perspective; a sense of humor almost always restores it. I love the delightful *Ellen Degeneres Show*. I find Ellen's sense of humor and attitude about life inspiring and uplifting, and I always feel better after watching it. I feel the same when I watch The *Oprah Show*; like Ellen, she also exudes joy, love, and positive enthusiasm. Also, think of the late president Ronald Reagan; he was popular and beloved partly because of his innate kindness with others, his fetching sense of humor, and his propensity to see the glass as half full—to focus on the positive and a hopeful future. And, the man who put millions of Americans to bed laughing for three decades, the late Johnny Carson, shared his cheerful heart and comedic acumen with us all and, according to Jay Leno, was the gold standard" in the industry. I agree. Making people laugh and being sanguine and optimistic are endearing and disarming qualities.

It was Norman Cousins, a noted journalist and author who, during a life-threatening illness, was able to achieve two hours of pain-free living for every ten minutes he devoted to laughter. In his renowned book, *Anatomy of an Illness,* he told about how he watched old comedies by the Marx Brothers and the Three Stooges and *Candid Camera* by the hour. He learned that laughter—hearty belly laughter—produced certain chemicals in the brain that benefit body, mind, and emotions.

According to researchers, laughter releases endorphins into the body that act as natural stress beaters. (One of my favorite remedies for stress is to watch a Steve Martin movie.) Laughter also aids most—and probably all—major systems of the body. A good laugh gives the heart muscles a good workout, improves circulation, fills the lungs with oxygen-rich air, clears the respiratory passages, stimulates alertness hormones that stimulate various tissues, and alters the brain by diminishing tension in the central nervous system. It also helps relieve pain and counteracts fear, anger, and depression—all of which are linked to physical illness and stress.

Scientific studies on the power of laughter were trumpeted on all the major television news stations. The studies disclose that one minute of laughter boosts the immune system for 24 hours! And one minute of anger suppresses immunity for 6 hours! The elixir of life—and the best way to soften your heart and diminish the wrinkles around your soul (and on your face!)—is hearty laughter. Laughter is a sterling stress buster and loving gift we can give ourselves and others in our lives. Laughter is calorie—and pain—free and costs nothing; the dividends are priceless.

Another superlative way to relieve pain and depression, improve circulation, reduce stress, and help balance your body and life is through massage.

15. SWEAT AND MASSAGE AWAY STRESS AND TENSION

Saunas, in one form or another, have been used across ages and oceans. Cultures around the world have recognized the relaxing benefits of rendered heat within a warm, welcoming space. From the Romans to the Japanese to the Scandinavians, heat therapy has been essential for the body to unwind from the stresses and hardships of daily life. For thousands of years, cultures throughout the world have enjoyed the many therapeutic benefits of saunas, from the elaborate bath/sauna/exercise complexes of the Romans, to the simple but effective "sweat lodge" structures of the Scandinavians and Native Americans. These cultures recognized the many therapeutic benefits of the sauna (i.e., rids body of toxins, aids weight loss, kills viruses), fully enjoying these benefits in a community setting.

In Finland, the sauna is a historic tradition. For over a thousand years, the sauna has been an important part of Finnish life and Finnish culture, cherished by every Finnish man, woman and child, according to Paavo Airola in his book *Health Secrets From Europe.* In fact, the sauna is credited for much of the rugged vitality and endurance—the sisu—of the Finnish people. In a country of approximately 5 million people, there are an estimated 700,000 saunas–one for every 7 people! Airola writes, "Most Finnish saunas are in separate buildings specially constructed for this purpose. Every farm has its own sauna, usually built on the shore of a lake or river. Most family houses in the city have saunas built on the lot, usually in the back yard."

Business meetings between strangers in Finland are often conducted in the soothing surroundings of the sauna, and it has been suggested that the combination of high heat and nakedness enabled the Finns to successfully negotiate the international trade minefields between East and West during the cold war. There is a saying in Finland that one must behave in the sauna just as in church. They consider taking saunas very sacred. What can we learn from the Finns about the benefits of saunas?

Sweating is not only an important part of our physical well-being, but in these modern times of water- and air-borne pollution, toxic chemicals, heavy metals and poor dietary and exercise habits, the therapeutic internal cleansing of regular sweating is critical to maintain a healthy body and mind. I wouldn't be without my sauna and I use it several times weekly, all year long.

The hot, dry air of the sauna is therapeutically different from the steam room sauna. The dry sauna causes profuse sweating, the air itself absorbing the sweat. But the water-saturated air of the steam room doesn't readily accept the sweat released by the body. The steam room makes you feel hotter because your sweat doesn't evaporate and carry away the heat. This raises a question: Is it better to be warm on the inside or sweaty on the outside?

That depends on what you want from either system. When exposed to heat of any kind, blood vessels in the skin dilate to allow more blood to flow to the surface. This activates the millions of sweat glands that cover the body. The fluid in the blood hydrates the sweat glands, which pour the water onto the skin's surface. As the water evaporates from the skin, it draws heat from the body; it's nature's cooling system.

Either the sauna or the steam room can be used to relax and unwind; however, the dry sauna clearly has more therapeutic benefits. For one thing, the dry sauna has an advantage over a steam room by helping to rid the body of more toxic metals picked up from our environment. Of course, the kidneys take out many of these toxins, but a daily sweat can help reduce the body's accumulation of lead, mercury, and nickel in addition to cadmium, sodium, sulfuric acid and cholesterol.

The sauna is also more beneficial over the steam room if weight loss is desired because of the energy expenditure. Compared to the steam room, the sauna places a greater demand on the body in terms of using up calories—therefore assisting in fat loss. The heart has to work harder to send more blood to the capillaries under the skin. The energy required for that process is derived from the conversion of fat and carbohydrates to calories. In addition, the sweat glands must work to produce sweat, which also requires energy and more calories. Studies show that a person can burn up to 300 calories during a sauna session, the equivalent of a 2–3 miles jog or an hour of moderate weight training.

Wet and dry saunas are available in many gyms and fitness centers throughout the country. Personally, I'd rather not sit or lie down on other peoples' sweat. Having my own sauna right in my home is one of the greatest blessings in my life because it keeps me detoxified, rejuvenated and youthful year-round.

For more information on the healing power of sweating and infrared saunas, please visit my website: **www.SusanSmithJones.com** and click on *Susan's Favorite Products*. Also, check out **www.healthmatesauna.com** or call: **1-800-946-6001**.

Taking regular saunas gives your skin a healthy, youthful glow…and so does massage. Keep in mind that skin is the human body's largest organ, accounting for 19 percent of our body weight and covering approximately twenty square feet, depending on our size. From the ancient Greek gymnasium and Roman baths to modern-day spas and health clubs, massage has been recognized for its health-enhancing effects. This age-old healing practice has enjoyed a renaissance in the last quarter century. Today, massage is a flourishing art form.

From infancy to old age, massage enhances general health and well-being. I've been getting and giving massages for 30 years, and for me it's the equivalent of a long nap, in terms of refreshment. Not only does it calm my nerves, release stress, and make me glow from the inside out, it energizes my body in a way that makes me feel youthful.

Therapeutic massage has numerous applications, variations, and techniques. Many of the therapeutic effects of massage recognized by personal and clinical experience over the years have been supported by scientific research. In addition to the commonly known benefits of relaxation and stress relief, new applications for therapeutic massage are surfacing in areas related to mental and emotional well-being, infant care, aging, athletics, and other special situations. Exciting new discoveries link touch and therapeutic massage to overall body rejuvenation/detoxification and improved immune system functions.

Therapeutic massage reduces stress and tension, improves circulation, relieves muscle spasms, helps to rid the body of toxins and retained fluids, and improves the skin. In terms of weight loss, the person massaging you is burning more calories than you are, but as your stress is massaged away, your hormones become more balanced, which aids in fat reduction. Some people claim it aids in cellulite reduction. While I've never seen any good studies to prove that, I have seen impressive results in clients. Best of all, I know that massage feels terrific. My favorite place to give or receive a massage is in a private place outdoors in nature. It could be on the deck of your home, in the backyard, or at a special resort.

16. ENJOY TIME IN NATURE

Being out in nature, where the air is filled with healthy negative ions, lifts the spirits, relaxes the body, and gives us a sense of well-being. The air all around us is electrically charged with positive and negative ions. Most of us live and work in environments dominated by technology—surrounded by computers, microwaves, air conditioners, heaters, TVs, and vehicular traffic. These and other "conveniences" of modern life emit excessive amounts of positive ions into the air we breathe, which can result in mental or physical exhaustion and affect overall wellness. But when you're in nature, especially surrounded by water—like the ocean or a stream or lake—or in a forest of green trees, negative ions abound. In fact, the revolving water generated by fountains creates negative ions that cause air particles to achieve electrical (ionic) balance.

One way to increase the negative ions in your environment is to surround yourself with fountains. I have them all over my home—in my gardens and in several rooms—running 24/7 except in the bedroom, where I prefer quiet when sleeping. Since ancient times, the sound created by moving or flowing water has been known to have great healing power. It has been said that the movement of water releases negative ions (chi energy) which, in turn, makes you feel refreshed, bringing peace to your heart and mind.

One of my favorite activities is hiking in the nearby Santa Monica Mountains early in the morning. When hiking you can take in a variety of terrain, flora, and fauna, while soaking up a wide range of sensations, sights, sounds, and scents as you move and work out your entire body. Hiking strengthens your body and feeds your soul, and you feel invigorated throughout the day.

We can learn so much from Mother Nature. She shows us the rhythm of the seasons and the balance of existence. She shows us the importance of times of withdrawal in attaining peace and serenity; the necessity of acceptance—flowing with the conditions of life; the wise use of energy and play; the true freedom that comes from lack of self-consciousness; and the strength that comes from being totally in the present.

One thing I know for sure. I always feel more positive and filled with gratitude when I spend quality time out in nature.

17. CULTIVATE AN ATTITUDE OF GRATITUDE

Choose to be positive and grateful every day. The link between mind and body has been contemplated since the time of Plato, but it's only recently that research has been done on the neurophysiology of the brain. Every thought transmits instructions to the body through some 70 trillion nerve cells, so when you think a negative thought, your immune system is immediately compromised. By the same token, when you think positive thoughts, your immune system is enhanced and your whole body benefits. Furthermore, an anxious or fearful mind instructs the body to be likewise—tense and nervous. A calm mind creates a calm body.

Keep your thoughts imbued with your highest vision of how you'd like to live and what you want to experience in life. In other words, visualize your goals and dreams. Dream big! Regardless of circumstances, always be persistent and keep the faith because you can create your heart's desires. You are full of infinite possiblilities; whatever you can imagine, you can accomplish. Paramahansa Yogananda once said the following: You can accomplish anything if you do not accept limitations… whatever you make up your mind to do, you can do. Similarly, in his books *Jonathan Livingston Seagull* and *Illusions,* author Richard Bach writes that you are never given a wish without also being given the ability to make it come true. And it was the mythologist Joseph Campbell who offered the following exquisite advice: Follow your bliss. When I pay attention to and honor the stirrings of my heart and soul, I look and feel younger. We age quickly when we live with regret instead of cultivating our highest visions and dreams.

So choose your thoughts wisely. A new report from the Mayo Proceedings suggests that individuals who profess pessimistic explanations for life events have poorer physical health and a higher mortality rate compared with either optimists or "middle-of-the-road" types, regardless of age or sex. In fact, every 10-point increase in the study's pessimism scores was associated with a 19 percent increase in the risk of death. Conversely, participants whose test scores indicated optimism had a survival rate significantly better than expected. The reason for this may be that pessimists may be more "passive" or have a "darker" outlook on life than other personality types, leaving them more prone to bad life events—such as illness, injury, and depression. The researchers concluded that pessimism itself is a "risk factor" for early death, and should be viewed in the same way as other risk factors, such as obesity, high blood pressure, or high cholesterol level.

When you find one thing, however small, to be thankful for and you hold that feeling for as little as 15 seconds, research reveals that many subtle and beneficial physiologic changes take place in your body, including the following four:

Health Benefits of Gratitude

1. Stress hormone levels of cortisol and norepinephrine decrease, creating a cascade of beneficial metabolic changes such as an enhanced immune system;

2. Coronary arteries relax, thus increasing the blood supply to your heart;

3. Heart rhythm becomes more harmonious, which positively affects your mood and all other bodily organs;

4. Breathing becomes deeper, thus increasing the oxygen level of your tissues.

If all of this happens when you focus for just 15 seconds on something that brings you pleasure, joy, or a feeling of gratitude, imagine what would happen to your health if you were able to cultivate grateful thoughts and feelings regularly, at least once per hour throughout each day of the year. The health benefits of gratitude (which is really the same thing as love) are an amazing example of how connected the bridge between the mind, body, and emotions really is and how simple it is to put this connection to work in your own life. But, as you well know, simple isn't necessarily easy. Like everything important in life, you must make a conscious choice and take action.

Gratitude (and appreciation) is a magnetic force that draws more good to each one of us. It's a dynamic spiritual energy that allows you to exert a powerful influence on your body, life, and world. Most importantly, it's a stellar stress-buster. What you think about consistently, you bring about in your life. Keep a gratitude journal and each day write down at least three things for which you are grateful. Focusing on the positive things, even during the most difficult times, is the perfect remedy to reduce and alleviate stress. And if you don't feel positive and grateful, "fake it until you make it," as the saying goes. In other words, "acting as if" will help you through many challenging times and carry you on to better times. It was Shakespeare who championed this sage advice in his immortal words in *Hamlet*: "Assume a virtue, if you have it not."

If there's one DVD movie that you'll want to own and watch often, I highly recommend *You Can Heal Your Life, The Movie* by Louise L. Hay & Friends. Are you in need something to empower and motivate you to enrich the quality of your life and bring your dreams and goals to fruition? Well, this entertaining and inspirational movie, based on the best-selling book of the same name, is the perfect ticket. Hosted by author and teacher Louise L. Hay, this film gives penetrating insights into Louise's fascinating personal story and shows how her views on self-esteem, abundance, and success were developed. It also reveals how she applies these concepts to her own emotional, spiritual, and professional life. For more information, or to order, please visit: **www.hayhouse.com** or call: **1-800-654-5126**.

One of the countless things I'm grateful for in my life is my friendships with others, including my dear friend Louise Hay. I treasure being surrounded by tenderhearted people.

18. HONOR FRIENDSHIPS WITH A TENDER HEART

I highly value and feel a great sense of gratitude for the love and support I receive from my friends, and for the opportunity to care deeply for others. The way to have a friend is to be one. Friends help sustain us when we're down, comfort us when we're sad, and offer counsel when we're confused. Friends are truly the best kind of wealth we can have—a wealth not calculated in numbers, but in the priceless value of love and kindness. Show comity, love, and appreciation for your friends. Never take your friends for granted. Friendship is as sacred a commitment as any: our friends are sent by God, so that we can help them and they can help us.

Often in today's society we are tempted to put our selfish interests first, before loyalty or integrity or commitment to higher values. Since what emanates from us will come back to us at some point, this is ultimately not a winning attitude. True friendship can be one of the rewards. The love shared between two people is the most precious gift we have. I appreciate this thought by T.S. Eliot who wrote: "What do we live for, if not to make life easier for one another." Jesus taught his followers to love one another. Paramahansa Yogananda gives us his sage, spiritual perspective in this quote: "It is God who comes to you in the guise of a true and noble friend to serve, inspire, and guide you." That's what my friendships do for me. They also teach me the importance of being kind and gentle with others. Gentleness and kindness usually ride tandem.

According to *Webster's* latest edition, gentle means kindly, mild, amiable, not violent or severe. It means compassionate, considerate, tolerant, calm, mild-tempered, courteous and peaceful. But I think that the best synonym for gentle is tender-hearted. I really like that word. And I love being around people who are tenderhearted.

To be treated with tenderheartedness, we must first offer that quality to other people. Respond to others exactly as you would want to be treated. No one likes to be rushed or belittled, ignored or unappreciated. Everyone likes kindness, patience and respect. *Ephesians* 4:32 advises, "Be kind to one another, tenderhearted, forgiving one another..." As my mom always taught me, simple and mellifluous words like "please" and "thank you" are always welcome and much needed in our stress-filled lives.

In the heart-warming movie, *Enchanted*, the princess, beautifully portrayed by Amy Adams, is a shining example of a tenderhearted person, someone you'd love to count as one of your friends.

Reaching out with a kind act or word of praise or appreciation can be so simple. Yet sometimes we assume that others "have it together," and do not need our kindness. Wouldn't it be better to move beyond our assumptions and to offer the kind of thoughtfulness we would appreciate receiving—a compliment, a smile, a hug, a pat on the shoulder, a note of thanks, or just a question that shows concern? If your kind gesture goes unnoticed or is refused, it doesn't matter, because in giving to another, you give to yourself. You'll feel better. Gandhi said that the pure loving kindness of one gentle soul can nullify the hatred of millions. Because we live in such a turbulent world, it's more important than ever for all of us to live more tenderheartedly. It will bring more joy and balance to our planet.

Another wonderful way to bring more joy and balance to your life and the world is through the companionship of animal friends, such as dogs, cats, horses, birds, rabbits, and fish. Studies show that people who live with pets are healthier than those who don't. Pet owners have lower cholesterol and triglyceride levels, and are less likely to suffer from nervousness, insomnia, stomachaches, headaches, and other minor health problems. New pet owners, especially dog owners, experience an increase in psychological well-being, self-esteem, and calmness. Consider opening your home to more animal friends.

19. MEDITATE AND LIVE WITH QUIET REVERENCE AND EQUANIMITY

Ralph Waldo Emerson knew the key to living with serenity and calmness. Meditation. It's a simple process of turning within and connecting with our own life force—our inherent, ever-present source of love, peace, joy, and guidance. Emerson offers us this sapient thought. "What lies behind us and what lies before us are small matters compared to what lies within us."

Take time each day to pray, meditate, talk to God, and simply spend a few minutes in silence. Studies have found lower rates of depression and stress among those who believe in God. If you are not religious, meditate. Prayer and meditation help us keep things in perspective, keep our minds calm and our lives balanced.

Practicing regular meditation is one of the best ways to bring stress hormone levels back to normal quickly, especially after an adrenaline-producing, cortisol-raising experience. I know of no more effective way to bring about relaxation than through meditation—turning inward in silence and reconnecting with the peace and calmness that's always within you. Featured in a *Time* magazine cover story (August 4, 2003, "The Science of Meditation"), meditation is being embraced around the world because of its numerous physiological, mental, emotional, and spiritual benefits.

When you think of meditation, you may envision crossed

legs and chants of "ommmm," but meditation can be anything that helps you focus your attention and increase your awareness of your body and the silence within you. Numerous scientific studies on meditation have shown it to cause a generalized reduction in many physiological and biochemical stress indicators, including decreases in heart rate, respiration rate, stress hormones, and pulse rate, and increases in oxygen consumption and slow alpha waves (a brain wave associated with relaxation). It is now being used successfully by people suffering from chronic pain and chronic conditions such as cancer and heart disease, as well as stress-related disorders, including abdominal pain, chronic digestive disorders, and ulcers.

For 35 years, I have been a disciplined meditator, and I teach workshops on the topic worldwide and work privately with individuals and families on simple ways to incorporate meditation into their lifestyle. For those of you who would like comprehensive information on meditation, its salutary benefits, and how to use it to reduce stress and achieve your goals, please refer to my audiobooks, *Choose to Live Peacefully* and *Wired to Meditate,* and my audio programs, *Celebrate Life!* and *EveryDay Health— Pure & Simple,* all available from my website or call: **1-800-843-5743**.

Nurture this inner peacefulness by bookending your day with quiet meditation for at least 10–15 minutes first thing in the morning and again before you go to sleep at night. This quietude will remind you that you can make the choice every day to live in the world, but not be caught up in the frenzy of it. If we have peace within ourselves, we don't have to make an effort to spread it; we radiate it to whomever comes into our presence. Choose to make peace your "default" position in life.

Part of the meditation process is focused deep breathing. In fact, conscious breath—inhaling and exhaling slowly and deeply—is itself a form of meditation. In addition to practicing deep breathing while meditating, take mini-breathing breaks throughout your day. While you're breathing, be sure to focus on your breath or a relaxing, peaceful, and joyful thought, and not on anything that might be stressful.

Another aspect of meditation and living a balanced, healthy, and joyful life is carving out moments of silence for yourself (as you do with meditation), even if it's only for a few minutes a day. Noise seems to part of our everyday lives—from the alarm clock in the morning and the traffic outside to the never-ending sounds of voices, radio and television, computers, and gardening equipment. Our bodies and minds appear to acclimate to these outside intrusions. Or do they?

The Committee on Environmental Quality of the Federal Council for Science and Technology found that "growing numbers of researchers fear the dangerous and hazardous effects of intense noise on human health are seriously underestimated." The late Vice President Nelson Rockefeller, when writing about the environmental crisis of our time, noted that when people are fully aware of the damage noise can inflict on man, "Peace and quiet will surely rank along with clean skies and pure waters as top priorities for our generation."

More recent studies, highlighted in the informative book *Save Your Hearing Now,* by Michael D. Swidman, M.D., FACS and Marie Moneysmith (isn't that a great name?), suggest that we pay the price for adapting to noise—higher blood pressure, heart rate and adrenaline secretion, heightened aggression, impaired resistance to disease, and a sense of helplessness. Studies indicate that when we can control noise, its effects are much less damaging.

I haven't been able to find any studies on the effects of quiet in repairing the stress of noise, but I know intuitively that most of us love quiet and need it desperately. We are so used to noise in our lives that silence can sometimes feel awkward and unsettling. On vacation, for instance, when quiet prevails, we may have trouble sleeping. But choosing times of silence can enrich the quality of our lives tremendously. If you find yourself overworked, stressed-out, irritated, tense, or out of balance, rather than heading for a coffee or snack break, maybe all you need is a silence break.

Everyone at some time has experienced the feeling of being overwhelmed by life. Everyone, too, has felt the need to escape, to find a quiet, secluded place to experience the peace of Spirit, to be alone with quiet thoughts. Creating times of silence in your life takes commitment and discipline. Most of the time, intervals of peaceful silence must be scheduled into your day's activities or you'll never have any.

Maybe you can carve out times of silence while at home where you can be without radio, television, telephones or voices. If you live in a family, maybe the best quiet time for you is early in the morning before others arise. In that silence, you can become more aware, more sensitive to your surroundings, and more in touch with the wholeness of life and your inherent inner guidance or intuition.

20. LISTEN TO YOUR INNER VOICE

Have you ever been thinking of someone you haven't heard from in a long time when suddenly that person called? Did you ever have the feeling that a friend was in trouble, and then contacted her and found out that she was, indeed? Or have you ever met someone and somehow known that this person was going to be your spouse? Some call it a sixth sense, a hunch, a gut feeling, going on instinct, or just knowing deep inside. Psychologists call it intuition—an obscure mental function that provides us with information so that we know without knowing how we know. I refer to it as God talking to us and giving us direction. It was Ralph Waldo Emerson who said: "Let us be silent that we may hear the whispers of God."

How tuned-in are you to this voice within? When you get a message, do you usually write it off as nothing? I have found from countless experiences that as we pay attention to our intuition and act on what we hear or feel, we reduce stress and create more balance in our lives. The key here is not just getting the message, but listening to it and acting on it. According to Nancy Rosanoff, author of *Intuition Workout,* one study asked divorced couples when they first realized the relationship wasn't going to work out, and an astounding *80 percent* replied, "before the wedding." Although something told them that the marriage was foolhardy, each couple stood together at the altar, either because they wished too strongly that their intuition was wrong, or they didn't identify the message as a kind of knowing they could trust.

So how can we develop the intuitive side of our being? The best way is just to sit still and listen. Turn within and pay attention. Too often we run away from ourselves, filling up our lives with constant, stress-filled activity. We don't take time to be still. Often creative geniuses report that their "real world" discoveries are nothing other than self-discoveries from a deep silence within. When someone asked William Blake where he got his ideas, he replied that he stuck his finger through the floor of heaven and pulled them down. Michelangelo spurned the congratulations that were proffered him after having turned a block of stone into a sculpture of a man by saying the man was in there all the time and just required a little help in getting out.

Franz Kafka wrote:

> There is no need to leave the house. Stay at your desk and listen. Don't even listen, just wait. Don't even wait, be perfectly still and alone. The world will unmask itself to you, it can't do otherwise. It will rise before you in raptures.

There is a profound benefit to hitting the pause button on your life every so often to create mini-respites, enabling you to connect with your inner silence and power.

Intuition can be nurtured in a variety of ways—through prayer, contemplation, walks in nature, or time spent alone gazing out a window or thinking. The more you act on your intuitive hunches, the stronger and more readily available they become. As you become more sensitive to your oneness with Spirit and life, you will become more intuitive. Part of receiving those inner messages clearly comes when you learn to give up the analyzing, reasoning, doubting, and limiting part of your mind. Practice makes perfect. And intuition is infallible when you anchor yourself in the consciousness of the Divine. In *The Tao of Pooh*, Benjamin Hoff shares:

> The masters of life know the Way. They listen to the voice within them, the voice of wisdom and simplicity, the voice that reasons beyond cleverness and

knows beyond knowledge. That voice is not just the power and property of a few, but has been given to everyone.

And it was Helen Keller who gave us the following sagacious advice: "The most beautiful things in the world cannot be seen or even touched. They must be felt with the heart."

How can you simplify your life so that what's really important—what's really essential to live fully and celebrate life—can be uncovered and nurtured? This brings us to the last tip for reducing stress and living a more balanced, joyful life.

21. SIMPLIFY YOUR PATH TO PEACE AND LOVE

Simplify! What a wonderful word and a powerful process. The recent death of a dear friend made me sit down this morning and think about life and about how I could choose to live more fully. The following words by Alfred D'Souze came to mind:

For a long time it had seemed to me that life was about to begin—real life. But there was always some obstacle in the way, something to be got through first, some unfinished business, time still to be served, a debt to be paid. Then life would begin. At last it dawned on me that these obstacles were my life.

This quote reminds me that sometimes our lives are so cluttered that it's difficult to see clearly. In the movie *Dances with Wolves,* I was deeply touched by the simplicity with which the Lakota Sioux people lived—able to gather all their belongings at a moment's notice and move on to another homeland. We are all trying to orchestrate the stresses, complexities and responsibilities of modern life. But much of the complexity we experience is, in fact, self-imposed. As we grow in self-awareness and live more internally, life gets simpler. Instead of getting our cues from the outside world, we listen for cues from our heart. Mahatma Gandhi encouraged each of us to: "Live simply, so that others may simply live." Jesus taught his followers not to be attached to material life, but instead to focus more on spiritual matters. He showed by example how to live a simple—but richly rewarding—life, unburdened by possessions.

Simplifying doesn't necessarily mean we have to restrict our activities, but it does mean uncluttering our lives so that we can put all our energy into activities we really care about. Activities, material things, and relationships are all time and energy consumers. Maybe it's time to take inventory of your life and weed out the superfluous. Being simple with life—not naive, but clear—allows us to experience the present fully and deeply.

Plato wrote, "In order to seek one's own direction, one must simplify the mechanics of ordinary, everyday life." I like that. To begin uncluttering your life, start with your home. Weed out everything you don't need, want, or use. Spend 15 minutes a day working on one area of your home, like a drawer or a closet. After your home is simplified, look at how you live, what you do, and how you spend your time. For example, look at all the foods you eat in one meal. It's hard to appreciate any one of them fully when there are so many mixed together. Similarly, you could have a fantastic collection of art objects in your home worth millions of dollars, but if there are too many, it is difficult to appreciate each piece fully. By the same token, if you have too many obligations, details and responsibilities, life loses its luster. Follow the recommendation given by Henry David Thoreau in his classic book, *Walden*, "Our life is frittered away by detail…Simplify, simplify."

Peace Pilgrim was another personification of simplicity. To the world, she may have seemed poor, walking penniless and wearing or carrying in her pockets her only material possessions. But she was indeed rich in blessings that no amount of money could buy—health, happiness, and inner peace. Peace Pilgrim knew that material things come and go, that we can all survive quite comfortably with very little. The quality of our lives isn't created outside ourselves. It comes from a healthy self-image, inner joy, and balance, and our relationship with the Divine. She wrote:

The simplified life is a sanctified life,
Much more calm, much less strife.
Oh, what wondrous truths are unveiled—

Projects succeed which had previously failed.

Oh, how beautiful life can be.

Beautiful simplicity.

In *Profound Healing,* one of the most inspiring books I've read on healing and living fully, author and dear friend Cheryl Canfield related a story about simplicity that her friend Peace Pilgrim told her. The story was about a woman whose house burned down. She and her husband had been living in a big home where they had raised their family. After the fire, they moved into a house more suitable for just the two of them. Peace attempted to offer a word of sympathy, but the woman interrupted her and said, "Now I'll never have to clean out those closets, and I'll never have to clean out that attic." After telling this story, Peace wondered aloud if it wouldn't have been wiser to have simplified her home before the fire.

There was a time in my life when I found great pleasure in collecting material things. I would delight in buying lots of clothes, shoes, appliances, electronics, gadgets, books, and cars until I got to the point where I was seeking fulfillment from what I collected rather than from within. In the pursuit of material possessions, I began to lose sight of the spiritual side of my nature through which all fulfillment, joy, peace, and happiness come. I was looking outward to my collection of stuff for my value and worthiness as a human being rather than looking within.

Fortunately, I discovered that it's not what the world holds for you that's important, but what you bring to the world. When I realized that, it became clear to me that I wanted to live more simply. Sure, I still buy clothes and other items, but more often I'm giving away things and finding ways to make my life less complicated.

When we have chaos, clutter, and imbalance in our lives, including in our homes, we feel stressed out and chaotic in our minds. Here is something I've done for years that might interest you. I invite a guest over to my house, at least weekly; it helps motivate me to clean my home and consistently get rid of clutter and the nonessentials. I also tell my guest he or she can have anything in the pile of stuff I'm giving away.

When making simple or complicated decisions or choices in my life, I often use "peace" and "love" as my barometers. I ask myself: "Will making this choice bring more peace into my life, or diminish my level of peace?" Put another way, in each situation, ask whether each of your thoughts, words, and deeds create a greater or lesser awareness of love and peace. Another valuable question I ask myself when I'm feeling stressed out about something: "Will this be an issue for me in six months?" Usually the answer is "no."

One of the most powerful life lessons I have come to understand in my life is the importance of simplifying outer thngs so that my inner life can take the driver's seat. Living an uncluttered life gives me time for the things I really care about, like time to think, to read, to walk in nature, to meditate and watch the sunrise or sunset. Through simplification, I am more clear-minded, and, I believe, a kinder, more sensitive person. When there is time to meditate, walk, read, reflect, think, pray, and be in the simplicity and beauty of nature, then life has a more natural flow, which is very much like meditation. Life becomes meditation. The divine becomes perfect simplicity.

Munificent with her love and kindness and inspiring with her compassion and optimistic attitude, my mom was my greatest teacher. One of the many lessons I learned from her was to "lighten up"—especially when life is difficult and pitches us curves. She'd often say to me, "This, too, shall pass." Mom was always right. To use a baseball analogy, with a little faith, trust, and patience, we can all hit home runs. Never let the fear of striking out keep you from playing the game and giving it your best, guided by your highest vision.

I want to close this part of the book by sharing with you a passage I read a few days ago in a wonderful out-of-print-book, *The Simple Life,* by Joan Atwater.

Our lives are over-burdened, and living often seems to us a terribly complicated affair. The problems of the world are so incredibly complex and we see that there are no simple answers. The complexity always leaves us with a feeling of helplessness and powerlessness. And still, amazingly enough, we go on, day by day, always half subconsciously yearning for something simpler, something more meaningful.

So how we look at our lives and living becomes tremendously important. It's up to us to bring this authenticity, this simplicity, this directness, this unburdened clarity into our looking. If such a thing as living life fully interests you, then it's up to you to learn about it and live it.

May you come to know and experience Love as your ever-present companion and beacon in your life's journey. Choose to embrace the fullness of life with élan and aplomb, and welcome a sacred balance. I salute your great adventure and wish you joy, peace, happiness, and vibrant health.

COMMITMENT-TIME

Here are some changes and choices I (you) will make this week, this month, and this year to support my goal of creating a renewed life of vitality and purpose. I now choose vibrant health and commit to living a balanced life.

THIS WEEK:

1. _____
2. _____
3. _____
4. _____
5. _____

THIS MONTH:

1. _____
2. _____
3. _____
4. _____
5. _____

THIS YEAR:

1. _____
2. _____
3. _____
4. _____
5. _____

PERSONAL NOTES AND MORE GOOD INTENTIONS

_____

_____

_____

_____

_____

_____

_____

_____

_____

_____

_____   _____

SIGN   **DATE**

> TWO ROADS DIVERGED IN A WOOD, *and I—I took the one least traveled by, and that has made all the difference.*
>
> — ROBERT FROST

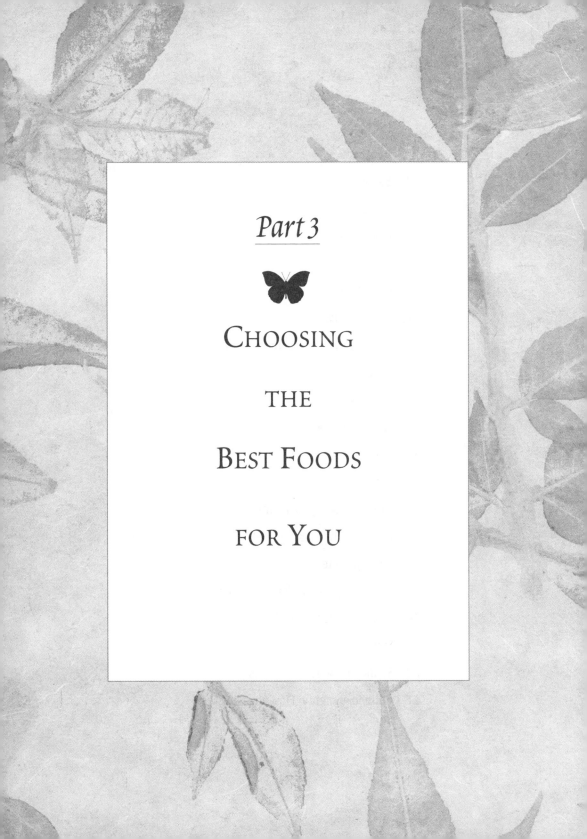

Part 3

CHOOSING

THE

BEST FOODS

FOR YOU

✓ 1. Avocado

✓ 2. Beans

3. Beets

✓ 4. Blueberries

✓ 5. Broccoli

✓ 6. Cantaloupe

✓ 7. Carrots & Parsnips

✓ 8. Citrus: Grapefruit, Lemon & Orange

9. Coconut

10. Flaxseed

✓ 11. Garlic & Onions

12. Kale

✓ 13. Kiwi

14. Nuts: Almonds & Walnuts

15. Peppers: Chilies & Red Bell

16. Pomegranate

17. Sea Vegetables: Dulse, Kelp & Nori

18. Spices: Cinnamon & Ginger

19. Spinach

20. Sunflower Seeds & Sprouts

21. Aphanizomnenon Flos-Aqua (AFA)

THE 21 "HOT" SUPERFOODS

Let food be your medicine and medicine be your food.

— HIPPOCRATES

As you know by now, for the past thirty-five years I have been a researcher, writer, teacher, lecturer, counselor and lifestyle coach, emphasizing holistic health, optimum nutrition, and the many benefits of living a balanced life. Many of you know me as the "Food Doctor," and you're aware that I have always looked to nature for answers on how to be my healthiest. I believe that God has provided us with every kind of food we need to nourish our bodies to create vibrant health right on into old age. This balanced, healthy lifestyle, particularly consuming a raw food diet, has allowed me to refrain from taking any prescription medication—something I count as a blessing indeed.

While the foods we eat are only one aspect of being healthy, diet is undeniably a very important component in overall health. A CNN Headline News report recently revealed that eight of the ten leading causes of death in North America are directly related to diet—a sobering statistic. And yet, we are all responsible for what we consume. Nobody shoves less-than-optimum food down our throats. Many of us choose the wrong foods every day, foods that were never intended for our bodies and which contribute to most common major diseases.

In Part 3 of this book, I will guide you on how to make the best choices from a selection of 21 "HOT" superfoods. What exactly can superfoods do? They can help reduce your risks of heart disease, hypertension, diabetes, obesity, Alzheimer's disease, arthritis, common forms of cancer, premature aging, vision problems and mental dysfunction. Not only that, these amazing foods can help increase your energy and vitality and provide a sense of empowerment over your body and life.

You'll learn the importance of selecting a variety of colorful, plant-based foods, preferably organically grown, as they do have more nutritional value. Each year, scientific studies disclose more about the active components of plant-based foods, called phytonutrients. These are chemical compounds in plants that act on human cells and genes to bolster your body's innate defenses against illness. Put simply, phytonutrients can save your life.

For decades my family, friends, and clients have asked my advice on the best natural remedies for a variety of physical conditions, ailments, and diseases. I recently recommended blueberries to a friend because they can increase brain longevity through their ability to help release dopamine in the brain. One of my clients is challenged with heart disease and cancer; on my list of foods to embrace and avoid, I recommended spinach and kiwi because of their high levels of disease-fighting antioxidants and phytonutrients, which are said to be excellent sources in battling those particular diseases. Finally, a participant in one of my workshops was concerned about fibroid tumors and I recommended pears because their high content of certain minerals and fibers is known to help prevent them.

While there are certainly more than 21 superfoods, I am going to share with you what I call my 21 "HOT" favorites—meaning that they are some of the best-of-the-best healing whole foods. For more information on these and additional salutary foods, please refer to my books, the 2-book Hay House series *The Healing Power of NatureFoods: 50 Revitalizing NatureFoods & Lifestyle Choices to Promote Vibrant Health* and *Health Bliss*.

Before I extol the virtues of these delectable foods, let me first introduce you to the ORAC analysis. ORAC refers to the "Oxygen Radical Absorbance Capacity," an analysis that is used to measure the total antioxidant power found in foods. The higher the ORAC score, the greater a food's antioxidant capacity. I refer to ORAC units simply as "anti-aging points." Researchers in the know suggest that we aim for 3,500 ORAC units per day. It might interest you to know, as well, that much of the antioxidant power in these colorful plant-based foods comes from the pigments in their skins.

OXYGEN RADICAL ABSORBANCE CAPACITY

VEGETABLES

ORAC units per 100 grams (about 3.5 ounces) of food for the following vegetables in descending order.

Food	ORAC units per 100 grams	Food	ORAC units per 100 grams
Kale	1,170	Red bell peppers	710
Spinach	1,260	Onions	450
Brussels sprouts	980	Corn	400
Broccoli florets	890	Eggplant	390
Beets	840	Carrots	210

FRUITS

ORAC units per 100 grams (about 3.5 ounces) of food for the following fruits in descending order.

Food	ORAC units per 100 grams	Food	ORAC units per 100 grams
Prunes	5,770	Plums	949
Raisins	2,830	Avocado	782
Blueberries	2,400	Oranges	750
Blackberries	2,036	Grapes	739
Cranberries	1,750	Cherries	670
Strawberries	1,540	Kiwi	602
Raspberries	1,220		

So let's begin with the first SuperFood...

1. AVOCADO −782 − 1/week

Often referred to as nature's butter, avocados are popularly known as the alligator pear because of the shape and rough skin of its most common variety, the Haas. Other types of avocado are larger in size and range in color from dark green to crimson. Avocados have more protein than any other fruit—approximately 2 grams in a 4-ounce serving.

Rich in phytochemicals, this fruit (yes, it is a fruit!) is the main ingredient in one of my favorite dishes—guacamole. Guacamole is scrumptious spread on whole grain bread or mashed into baked russet, yam, or sweet potatoes (instead of butter or margarine). You can even use it as a great hydrating facial mask (see Consider This, below). By weight, avocados have about a quarter of the calories of total fat of dairy butter. And ounce for ounce, they provide more heart-healthy monosaturated fat, vitamin E, folate (the plant source of folic acid), potassium and fiber than other fruits. In fact, four ounces, about one-half of a medium-size avocado, provides 500 mg. of potassium and more than 16 percent of the RDA of folate; it also supplies 10 percent or more of the RDA for iron, and vitamins C, E, and B-6.

Avocados are also rich in two phytochemicals: beta-sitosterol, an important phytochemical linked with lower cholesterol levels; and glutathione, an antioxidant that may offer protection against several cancers.

According to Susan Bowerman, R.D., a registered dietitian at the University of California at Los Angeles Center for Human Nutrition, avocados also exceed other fruits as a source of the potent antioxidant lutein. This antioxidant may help prevent cardiovascular disease such as atherosclerosis (hardening of the arteries) as well as prevent prostate cancer. In addition, lutein protects your eyes from cataracts and from age-related macular degeneration.

If all of this doesn't get you excited about avocados, maybe this will. World renowned nutrition expert David Heber, M.D., Ph.D., says in his insightful book, *What Color Is Your Diet?*, that avocados were known as "testicle fruit" to the ancient people of Central and South America. This delicious fruit also had a reputation as an aphrodisiac (I bet I have your attention now).

Avocados should always be eaten raw, since they have a bitter taste when cooked. A medium-sized California avocado contains about 30 grams of fat—almost twice as much as its Florida cousin—and more calories than any other fruit. Because of the high fat content (albeit healthy fat), if you wish to lose weight, limit your consumption to no more than one avocado per week. Avocados start to ripen only after being cut from the tree. Mature fruit can be left on the tree for six months without spoiling. Once picked, it will ripen in a few days.

> **CONSIDER THIS:** For a superb hydrating and rejuvenating facial mask, mash half an avocado and spread it on your face and neck. Relax for 15 to 60 minutes (on your bed, if possible), then wash it off. You'll feel and see the difference in your skin.

2. BEANS — Red Beans

Here is a food that certainly fits the superfood category. Legumes include fresh beans like peas, green beans and lima beans as well as lentils, chickpeas, black beans, pinto, navy, and red beans, and the whole dried bean family. Beans are not just a great source of fiber and protein; they also pack a powerful antioxidant punch. Vegetarians have long counted on beans as a replacement for protein-rich meat. The disease-preventing fiber and significant amount of protein in beans will also keep you satiated. Surprisingly, however, few scientists had bothered to see if beans contained antioxidants—free radical–destroying substances believed to help fight heart disease, cancer and more—until recently.

Dried beans are particularly rich in antioxidants called flavonoids, the ones found in green and black tea. The darker the bean, the more flavonoids it boasts. In other words, black beans have the most, then red, yellow, and finally white. The antioxidants are found in the bean coat which is where bean colors are also found.

Also, most beans are an excellent source of magnesium. Consuming magnesium can lower the risk of developing type 2 diabetes by up to 30 percent, as demonstrated in numerous studies involving thousands of women. More than 93 million women in the United States have type 2 diabetes.

Most beans are about 1 percent fat, while the soybean is about 18–20 percent fat, of which 15 percent is saturated, 23 percent monosaturated, and 58 percent polyunsaturated. The primary isoflavones in soy, genistein and daidzein, may help prevent cancer. However, one study found that anasazi, brown, black, navy, pinto and turtle beans contain about as much as or more genistein than soybeans (*Journal for Alternative Complementary Medicine.* 1997; 3:7–12).

Whether canned or fresh, beans are a great addition to toss in a salad or add to chili and pasta. If you choose canned beans, it's important to cut down on the salt content, so always put the beans in a strainer and rinse them with cool water, thus eliminating about 40 percent of the salt. Hummus, one of my favorite foods, is made from chickpeas (also known as garbanzo beans). I also sprout beans so I can create raw food hummus and other tasty treats. You can even grind dry beans (or grains) into healthy flour using the Kitchen Mill™ (visit my website, click on *Susan's Favorite Products,* then on Blendtec, or call **1-800-253-6383**). It takes little extra effort, and the enhanced flavor of the freshly ground beans or grains is something I always appreciate.

One last note regarding beans. It is indeed true that beans can cause flatulence. This is because bacteria attack the indigestible matter that remains in the intestine. The following remedies may work for you:

- Canned beans and mashed beans are less gas producing.

- If you eat beans frequently in small amounts, your body will become accustomed to them and you'll reduce any digestive problems.

- Soak beans before cooking, rinse and drain, add fresh water, and then boil them for two to three minutes. Turn off the heat and let them soak for a few hours. Rinse and drain again, add fresh water, and continue cooking per your recipe. This boiling and soaking releases a large percentage of the indigestible carbohydrate in the beans, making them easier to digest.

- Pressure-cooking beans also reduces their gas-producing qualities.

Being one who always looks for the positive, I figure that if you are adding to the "wind" or "breeze" in your environment, think of it as a splendid opportunity to spend some quality time alone. And, if you are a live-food cuisine enthusiast, you'll be happy to learn that the process of sprouting raw beans and lentils reduces their flatulence-factor.

> **CONSIDER THIS:** From the largest antioxidant study in history, the U.S. Department of Agriculture (USDA) has produced a list of the twenty most antioxidant-rich foods. The study examined more than one hundred types of fruits, vegetables, berries, nuts and spices. Winners included artichokes, russet potatoes and ground cloves, among other shockers, as top food sources of antioxidants. In the end, small red beans took the top spot, narrowly beating out wild blueberries as the food with the highest concentration of disease-fighting, anti-aging compounds per serving. It is believed that antioxidants—non-vitamin nutrients that abound in some foods—may benefit the body by providing protection against oxidation, a process that may be linked to conditions such as cancer, heart disease, and accelerated aging.

Found most often in colorful produce (plant-based foods), antioxidants are rarely found in animal products. In the USDA study published recently in the Journal of Agricultural and Food Chemistry, here's the full list of the top twenty, starting with the richest source of antioxidants and continuing in descending order. Notice how many of them are beans.

1. Small red beans
2. Wild blueberries
3. Red kidney beans
4. Pinto beans
5. Blueberries (cultivated)
6. Cranberries
7. Artichokes (cooked)
8. Blackberries
9. Prunes
10. Raspberries
11. Strawberries
12. Red Delicious apples
13. Granny Smith apples
14. Pecans
15. Sweet cherries
16. Black plums
17. Russet potatoes (cooked)
18. Black beans (dried)
19. Plums
20. Gala apples

3. BEETS

The sweet taste of the highly versatile beet belies its calorie content—a small beet has only 22 calories. These beautiful ruby-red root veggies are also a good source of folate, which is an important B-vitamin that protects against heart disease and cancer. One cup of the beet tops (the leafy green part), if eaten young and green, supplies 35 mg of vitamin C, 720 IU of vitamin A, 160 mg of calcium, 2.5 mg of iron, and a whopping 1,300 mg of potassium. My favorite way of utilizing the nutritious tops is by juicing them.

According to folklore, beets were believed to possess curative powers for headaches and other painful conditions. Even today, some health practitioners recommend beets to help prevent cancer and bolster immunity. I also suggest using raw beet juice to speed convalescence and as a good overall body detoxifier and rejuvenator.

Antioxidants recently discovered in beets show promise for preventing heart disease, although research is preliminary. According to a study published in 2001 in the *Journal of Agricultural Food Chemistry,* betanin, one of these antioxidants, inhibited oxidation of LDL ("bad") cholesterol. This effect was shown in a test tube, but the researchers also found that people were able to absorb the antioxidants by consuming beet juice. And here's another reason to eat beets. According to a recent animal study, consumption of beets significantly slowed the growth of skin and lung tumors.

There are so many ways to enjoy beets. They can be boiled and served as a side dish, pickled and eaten as a salad or condiment, or used as the main ingredient in borscht, a popular Eastern European cold summer soup. The most nutritious part of the vegetable, beet greens, can be cooked and served like spinach or Swiss chard or, as mentioned above, juiced with other vegetables such as carrots, celery, cucumbers and spinach. One word of warning, however: consuming beets may temporarily turn your urine and stools pink or even red. This is a harmless condition that occurs when betacyanin, the red pigment in beets, passes through the digestive system without being broken down. The urine and stools usually return to their normal colors after a day or two.

> **CONSIDER THIS**: For a tasty and colorful beet boost to my diet, I use BeetMax™ several times weekly in a variety of recipes, including to make a healthy, fast juice. It is a concentrated beet juice powder that is convenient to use and absolutely delicious. This product has the following properties: it is made from certified organic beets; it is a low temperature drying process that retains critical heat-sensitive nutrients and living enzymes; it has no sweeteners or artificial ingredients; it mixes easily with water to make a rich, nutritious juice. Offered exclusively through Hallelujah Acres (**www.Hacres.com** or **1-800-915-9355**), it is made using a proprietary dehydration process which is capable of dehydrating juice to a powder with minimum degradation of color, flavor, aroma, enzymes, and nutrition. (I also recommend their BarleyMax™ and CarrotMax™ powders. Mixing the three together makes a delicious, quick, and rejuvenating drink.)

4. BLUEBERRIES

Known as an excellent laxative, blood cleanser and antioxidant, blueberries are the only food that has been shown to not just prevent, but actually reverse abnormal physical and mental decline. Native to North America, blueberries have been part of the human diet for more than 13,000 years and rank among the best foods you can eat. I recommend eating them several times a week, fresh when you can get them, or in the winter, substitute frozen. I always have frozen organic blueberries on hand and use them liberally in my smoothies.

Despite their small size, one cup of blueberries contains almost 4 grams of fiber and only 80 calories. A whole pint gives you about 180 calories, so they're a dieter's best friend. Like all other foods, the calories in blueberries come from their macronutrients—56 grams of carbohydrate, 1.5 grams of fat, and 2.7 grams of protein. But it is blueberries' micronutrient content that packs the most impressive wallop.

Referred to as the "brain berry," blueberries are packed with red pigments, or anthocyanins, that have been linked to prevention—and even reversal—of age-related mental decline, and have anti-cancer effects. They are one of the most potent antidotes to oxidate stress, a process that ages you. The anthocyanins in blueberries appear to be responsible (according to a study released in 2002 by Tufts University in Boston). In fact, this study indicates that blueberries can reverse the harmful effects of aging on the neuronal signals in the brain—signals that are essential to memory. This research suggests that blueberries in the diet may also help in the fight against developing Alzheimer's disease. Nearly half the women over the age of 85 in the United States have this debilitating disease. "The research on blueberries and brain function is still in the very early stages," says Jeffrey Blumberg, Ph.D., professor at the Friedman School of Nutrition Science and Policy at Tufts University. "But it may very well pan out that they can prevent degeneration of the brain as we age." So why not enjoy them as a regular feature in your diet now?

Here's another reason to get acquainted with these little blue jewels. The flavonoids in blueberries—catechin, epicatechin, myricetin, quercetin, and kaempferol—are a mouthful of strangely spelled words, but more importantly, they are extremely valuable for superior health. Blueberries are to fruit what the next superfood, broccoli, is to vegetables. You would be hard-pressed to find any higher praise than that!

> **CONSIDER THIS:** You can make the most scrumptious "ice cream" by putting frozen blueberries and another frozen fruit of your choice, such as bananas, raspberries, papaya, or mangoes, through your Champion Juicer. It's just frozen fruit so it's very healthy; it takes only a few minutes to make and, depending on the fruit you use with the blueberries, it is as beautiful to eat as it is satisfying for any sweet tooth.

5. BROCCOLI

A supreme superfood, it is difficult to overstate broccoli's healing powers. Like other cruciferous vegetables (cabbage, cauliflower, and Brussels sprouts), broccoli has been proven effective in helping to prevent breast, colon, esophageal, and lung cancers in addition to heart disease and a host of other serious conditions. Two powerful cancer-fighting substances in this perfect food are sulforaphane and indole-3-carbinol. Sulforaphane gives cancer-causing chemicals a one-two punch: first, it destroys any carcinogenic compounds that you've ingested; second, it creates enzymes that eat up any carcinogens left over from that reaction.

Sulforaphane also kills the bacteria H. pylori, which causes ulcers and greatly increases the risk of gastric cancer, according to a recent study from Johns Hopkins University. A recent study in the *Journal of Nutrition* reveals that sulforaphane may also block the late stages of breast cancer cell growth. Indole-3-carbinol helps your body metabolize estrogen, potentially warding off breast cancer, a theory supported by epidemiological and clinical studies.

In addition to being a superlative cancer-buster, this tasty superfood is also a good source of beta carotene, calcium, magnesium, vitamin B-3, vitamin B-5, vitamin C, potassium, folate, chlorophyll and fiber. And the fiber in broccoli (4 grams in 1 cup) slows your body's release of blood sugar, helping to provide long-lasting energy. Very low in calories and nutrient-dense, this cruciferous vegetable may also inhibit the herpes simplex virus from reproducing. A substance called 13C, found in broccoli and related veggies, was found to be effective even though the herpes strain tested is resistant to current drugs.

I eat broccoli raw, lightly steamed, or juiced, and also in the form of sprouts, which magnifies broccoli's potent healing powers. To reap all of these powerful benefits of broccoli, or other cruciferous vegetables, be sure to have at least three to five half-cup servings of these veggies daily.

> **CONSIDER THIS:** Broccoli stalks are perfect to juice or even grate to add to a coleslaw salad along with cabbage and carrots.

6. CANTALOUPE

One of my favorite fruits, cantaloupe is an excellent cleanser and rehydrator because of its high water content. Like all melons, for easy digestion and maximum benefit, eat cantaloupe alone. This beautiful fruit contains lots of zinc, which is important for the prostate gland. Instead of your midmorning or midafternoon coffee or soda (and donut or cookie), eat half a cantaloupe, which makes a great snack and contains more vitamins A and C than an equal amount of just about any other fruit.

This sweet, succulent, and gorgeous fruit is also a power-house of potassium with one-quarter of a cantaloupe offering between 800 and 900 mg. That's one-quarter of your daily potassium requirements! (1 cup lima beans has 950 mg; 1 cup tomato sauce has 900 mg; 1 medium banana has about 450 mg).

According to new research, if you're not getting enough potassium, you could be putting yourself at risk for a stroke. Scientists tracked 5,600 adults for four to eight years and found that those who didn't eat enough potassium-rich foods were 1.5 to 2.5 times more likely to suffer from a stroke, even if they were on medications to help prevent stroke.

I bring cut-up chunks of cantaloupe for snacking when I fly or on lengthy, energy-draining car trips. It also makes the perfect food to eat exclusively throughout the day (mono diet) as a great detoxifier and rejuvenator once a month.

> **CONSIDER THIS:** If you can find organic cantaloupe, wash the skin and juice everything (along with a few sprigs of fresh mint) for a nutrient-rich, skin-enhancing, and delicious beverage.

7. CARROTS & PARSNIPS

Carrots are a stellar detoxifier and an excellent food for the health of the liver and digestive tract, registering 210 on the ORAC unit score for vegetables. Naturally sweet, they make an ideal high-fiber, low-calorie snack food. Those baby carrots you find already peeled and packaged in your grocery store are not really baby carrots, but simply prepared to look that way.

I'm sure you've heard that old wives' tale about the benefits of carrots for your eyes. Well, there's some truth to that. Carrots contain a broad mix of carotenoids, including lutein and zeaxanthin, which help prevent cataracts, macular degeneration, and night blindness. In fact, it may be possible to delay the development of night vision disturbances in later life by eating a wide variety of orange vegetables, especially carrots. Orange vegetables all contain vitamin A, and the more vitamin A you have in your body, the more rhodopsin you produce. Rhodopsin is a purple pigment that the eye needs in order to see in dim light. Carrots also contain additional antioxidants, including alpha-carotene, which fights cancer and heart disease. One of the reasons they are deemed a heart-healthy food is because they are rich in calcium pectate, a soluble fiber that lowers cholesterol.

One study found that a high intake of foods containing beta-carotene (one of the disease-fighting carotenoids) lowered the risk of breast cancer in certain populations of women. Another study found that a high intake of raw vegetables was associated with a decreased risk of breast cancer.

Although I prefer raw carrots, they are in fact one of those rare foods that increase in nutritional value when cooked because cooking breaks down the tough cellular walls that encase the beta-carotene. To convert beta carotene to vitamin A, the body needs at least a small amount of fat, because vitamin A is soluble in fat, not water. For that reason, I eat carrots with a little healthy fat such as avocado, nuts or seeds or flax oil (often combined in a salad). Grated carrots hold an esteemed place of honor in most of my salads that are topped with a healthy dressing. Eat some baby carrots right out of the fridge with a low-fat dip—a great way to get a bounty of health benefits.

Beware of a certain carrot quirk, though. My friends all know when I've been juicing carrots to mix with my other green vegetables as my skin turns a faint shade of orange-yellow. This condition, known as carotenosis, is most common in children but also appears in adults. It's harmless—so don't worry if you discover a color change in your skin. All you have to do is simply stop eating carrots for a few days and then you can begin enjoying them again, in moderation. For a delicious Carotenoid Cocktail, juice the following ingredients together and relish every sip: 3 carrots, 1 tomato, ½ cup red bell pepper, and 1 cup spinach.

CONSIDER THIS: As mentioned in the section on beets, CarrotMax™ (available through Hallelujah Acres, **www.Hacres.com**) is a fast and delicious way to get the benefits of carrot juice when you don't have time to make juice. The low temperature drying process of the powder retains the critical heat-sensitive nutrients and living enzymes.

PARSNIPS. This vegetable is from the same family as carrots and, surprisingly, tastes just as sweet. In fact, they even look like white/yellow carrots and have a sweet, nutty flavor that goes well with other vegetables in soups or stews. Low in calories, they can also be served as a side dish instead of potatoes or other starchy foods. I've read that they are too fibrous to eat raw; don't believe it. They can be juiced or grated and added to salads. In fact, I make a salad of grated parsnips and carrots and add a couple ounces of organic raisins and an ounce of sunflower seeds or ground flaxseed or chopped walnuts or almonds—all tossed together with some light, fresh dressing.

Cucumbers, watermelon, red bell peppers, flaxseed, avocado, and parsnips could each be nicknamed "the beauty food." The nutritional components in parsnips help strengthen hair and nails and improve skin quality. People suffering from acne or other skin disorders will appreciate parsnips' unique balance of potassium, phosphorus, sulfur, silicon, chlorine, and vitamin C, all of which benefit the skin. A half-cup serving has only 60 calories and is high in fiber; it also provides 300 mg of potassium and between 10 and 20 percent of the daily requirements of vitamin C and folate. Their chlorine and phosphorus levels improve function in the lungs and the bronchial tubes. Parsnips have been used as a diuretic, an anti-arthritic agent, and for detoxifying. I also recommend parsnip juice to help dissolve gall and kidney stones.

The parsnips available in supermarkets are often too old and flabby and rarely worth purchasing. No wonder so few people use them today. A parsnip that is allowed to remain in the ground at least two weeks past the first frost is unbelievably sweet and satisfying, so they're best in the late fall and winter. Select ones about the size of a medium carrot; reject any that are covered with roots or are soft and shrunken.

Most parsnips are sold with the tops removed; if the tops are still attached, cut them off before storing them so they don't draw moisture from the roots. Look for straight, smooth-skinned roots that are a tan or creamy-white color, firm and fresh-looking, without gray, dark, or soft spots. They can be kept for a few weeks in the refrigerator. So, the next time you buy carrots or other vegetables for juicing, mix it up. Add half a pound of parsnips and enjoy their sweet nutrition.

> **CONSIDER THIS:** I mash steamed parsnips just as I do russet or Yukon gold potatoes. Add some roasted garlic for an unforgettable, healthy side dish.

8. CITRUS: GRAPEFRUIT, LEMON & ORANGE

As with all other citrus fruits, grapefruit is rich in vitamin C and potassium and very low in calories. A cup of fresh squeezed grapefruit juice has 95 mg of vitamin C, more than 100 percent of the RDA. This fresh raw juice eases constipation and improves digestion by increasing the flow of gastric juices. One whole grapefruit has only 100 calories and it makes a perfect snack food. The red and pink varieties are high in beta carotene and lycopene. Deep inside the white rind and membranes of this fruit lies a miraculous group of plant compounds—bioflavonoids, citric acids, and pectins. Lemons and oranges are bursting with these compounds as well.

These plant compounds protect against cancer and heart disease. Grapefruit pectin reduces the accumulation of athero-sclerotic plaque in patients afflicted with atherosclerosis and strengthens blood vessels and capillaries. Some people with rheumatoid arthritis, lupus, and other inflammatory disorders find that eating grapefruit daily seems to alleviate their symptoms. This may occur because plant chemicals block the prostaglandins that cause inflammation.

Grapefruit is definitely a multiple-benefit fruit. Do you need to lose weight? Make grapefruit your first course to help prevent overeating. The pectin content of grapefruit reduces appetite by slowing the emptying of the stomach. Suffering from a cold? Grapefruit juice helps reduce fever and soothes coughs and sore throats. If I ever feel a cold coming on, which is rare, I blend one peeled grapefruit with some water, fresh ginger, and cayenne pepper, drink the liquid and feel it go to work in minutes. Trouble sleeping? Consumed at night, grapefruit juice promotes sleep and alleviates insomnia. And remember: think pink. Pink and red varieties are far more nutritious than white grapefruit.

CONSIDER THIS: Put some essential oil of grapefruit (not for internal use) on the inside of your wrists and a dab behind each ear to help keep you from overeating. When purchasing grapefruit or lemons, look for the heavier, smooth- and thin-skinned ones as they have the most juice and the most bang for the buck.

LEMON. Although acid to the taste, the juice of a lemon is a great alkalizer for the body. When our bodies are too acid, our immune systems are compromised and our energy abates. Of all the citrus fruits, lemon is the most potent detoxifier. According to Steve Meyerowitz in his book *Power Juices Super Drinks,* lemon kills some types of intestinal parasites such as round-worms, and also dissolves gallstones. Limonene, the volatile oil responsible for the distinctive lemon aroma and an oil that can irritate the skin in susceptible persons, even helps treat some forms of cancer such as breast cancer.

Taken in the morning on an empty stomach (and diluted with water), lemon juice is known to improve liver function and has been used to help eliminate kidney stones. The organic acids in all citrus fruits stimulate digestive juices and relieve constipation. Added to water or fresh juice, lemon juice helps relieve colds, coughs, and sore throats. If you have dry mouth, licking a lemon or sipping unsweetened diluted lemon juice can stimulate saliva flow. Too much lemon juice, however, if left on the teeth, can erode tooth enamel, so rinse out your mouth with pure water or brush your teeth after consuming lemon juice.

Lemons contain the highest amounts of both vitamin C and citric acid, more than any other citrus fruit; the juice of a medium lemon has more than 30 mg of vitamin C. They also offer potassium, magnesium, calcium and pectin. When a recipe calls for fresh lemon zest, which is the grated outer peel, make sure its from an organic lemon or else it might have been waxed or sprayed with chemicals. I go through 3-4 lemons a day; my favorite is the Meyer lemon. Each morning upon awakening, I drink the juice of one half lemon stirred into a large glass of hot water; I add a half lemon when making fresh vegetable juices—peel and all; I use it in salad dressings; I sprinkle it on vegetables. Fresh lemon juice improves the flavor of many vegetables, especially those that contain sulfur compounds, such as broccoli. Concerned about weight? Lemon juice is a perfect nonfat alternative to butter, oil dressings and rich sauces. Invest in a good citrus juicer; it's inexpensive, user-friendly, and very practical.

CONSIDER THIS: I love lemon zest on almost anything. Using a microplane, grate some of the yellow lemon peel (zest) on any dish for a fresh, citrusy flavor.

ORANGE. Long considered a favorite breakfast food, fresh orange juice, or the whole orange, is a potent source of vitamin C. The recommended daily allowance (RDA) for Americans is 90 mg a day for adult males and 75 mg for adult females, although I recommend a more optimal intake of dietary vitamin C of 350 mg or more from food.

According to research, up to a third of us consume less than 60 mg of C daily—well below the RDA. Among other functions, vitamin C is essential for the formation of collagen—the connective tissue matrix within our bones. A single navel orange, at only 64 calories, provides 83 mg of vitamin C as well as folate, thiamine, and potassium plus citrus flavonoids, which are found in the fruit's tissue, juice, pulp and skin. One of the flavonoids, hesperidin, is a superb antioxidant and antimutagenic. The latter refers to its ability to prevent cells from mutating and initiating one of the first steps in the development of cancer and other chronic diseases. Hesperidin also works to revive vitamin C after it has quenched a free radical. In other words, the hesperidin strengthens and amplifies the effect of vitamin C in your body. In one clinical trial, orange juice was shown to elevate HDL cholesterol ("good") while lowering LDL ("bad") cholesterol.

The sunny orange also provides beta-cryptoxanthin, a carotenoid that may help prevent colon cancer. Nobiletin, a flavonoid found in the flesh of oranges, may have anti-inflammatory actions. You're probably familiar with the pectin in oranges, the dietary fiber that's so effective it helps to reduce cholesterol. It is present in large amounts in the white lining of citrus fruit. An easy way to increase your pectin intake is to eat the white pith. I always eat the "white stuff" on the inside of orange or tangerine rinds, scooping up a little of the orange color as well to boost my limoene intake. Limoene is an oil that may help treat some forms of cancer such as breast cancer. Oranges are a delicious snack and a flavorful ingredient in salads. Canned oranges lose most of their vitamin C and some minerals during processing and are usually packed in high-sugar syrups. Go for fresh!

Fresh juice is a snap to make. You can literally juice an orange in seconds with a citrus juicer, although I prefer to put the entire *organic* orange through my more powerful juicer to extract the most nutrients from this vital and delicious fruit.

Since this drink is so popular, let's get more specific. OJ is a superb source of folate, vital to a healthy pregnancy to reduce risk of birth defects. Folate is also important for a healthy heart and helps prevent anemia. OJ contains potassium, which helps keep blood pressure down, and vitamin C, linked to lower rates of cancer. Each 8-ounce cup (110 calories) contains 11 percent of your daily need for potassium. So drink up. You might also enjoy the taste of OJ mixed with some pomegranate juice or coconut milk as described below.

CONSIDER THIS: Blood oranges are a beautiful (and I mean beautiful!) alternative to navel and juice oranges. They are nutritious, delicious, and colorful, with hues of orange, pink, purple and red inside. Make juice with blood oranges that will treat your taste buds to something extraordinary and unforgettable.

9. COCONUT

Coconut butter (also referred to as coconut oil) has been used as a food and a medicine since the dawn of history. Ayurveda (the medicine of India) has long advocated its therapeutic and cosmetic properties. Unlike the cooked, clogging, cholesterol-laden, saturated fats found in meats and dairy products, coconut butter is a raw saturated fat containing mostly medium-chain fatty acids (MCFA's) which the body can metabolize efficiently and convert to energy quickly. Coconut butter contains no cholesterol and does not elevate bad (LDL) cholesterol levels.

By weight, coconut butter has less calories than any other fat source. The MCFA's in coconut butter possess incredible properties. Bruce Fife, ND, author of the terrific book *The Coconut Oil Miracle,* has written: "Coconut oil is, in essence, a natural antibacterial, antiviral, and antifungal." Added regularly to a balanced diet, it may help lower cholesterol by promoting its conversion into pregnenolone. Pregnenolone is the precursor to many hormones, including progesterone. Rich in magnesium, potassium, zinc, folate and vitamin C, coconut also helps regulate thyroid function.

Coconut water and coconut milk are marvelous, healthful beverages. My favorite part of the coconut is the liquid that develops naturally inside the coconut, called "coconut water." Technically speaking, it is different from coconut milk, although the two terms are often interchanged. "True coconut milk is a manufactured product made from the flesh of the coconut. It is prepared by mixing water with grated coconut, squeezing and extracting the pulp, leaving only the liquid," writes Fife. The coconut milk is higher in fat than the coconut water, containing between 17 and 24 percent fat.

Next to purified, filtered water, coconut water is my favorite beverage. Filling the cavity inside the young coconut, this luscious liquid is colorless but slightly cloudy and sweet-tasting. Coconut milk, on the other hand, resembles cow's milk; it is pure white and is not sweet unless sugar has been added. Available in most grocery and health food stores, you can enjoy coconut milk by the glass, use to replace cow's milk, add to smoothies, pour over cereal or fresh fruit, or add it to other juices or tea. Try blending coconut milk, orange juice, and some fresh fruit. The coconut milk gives the juice a delicious creamy taste and texture. As for the coconut water, always go fresh! Look for the young, white coconuts in your health food store, cut off the top, and pour this salubrious liquid into your favorite glass. Several times weekly, I savor a tropical treat of coconut water, often combined with some fresh lemon juice. You can also add this coconut water to other juices.

Another versatile product of this asymmetrical, humble-looking nut, coconut butter can be eaten straight or blended into a salad dressing, mixed into a smoothie, or incorporated into raw food cuisine. It can also be used as a skin lotion. It's very effective against dry skin and is ideal for massage. This is the main moisturizer I've used on my skin for years and on my hair as a bi-weekly deep conditioner. Coconut butter should be stored in a cool, dark area. Most butters and oils are light-sensitive so make sure it is in a dark container to insure no light penetrates and damages the oil. Always choose a raw, cold-pressed coconut butter, never heated.

> **CONSIDER THIS**: Every week or two, I put coconut butter on my hair for an excellent deep conditioner. Time permitting, I'll sit in the sauna or, at least, put on a shower cap to help the coconut butter penetrate my hair shaft more completely. Wash it out and you'll see a beautiful shine and silky softness to your hair.

10. FLAXSEED

Often referred to as "nutritional gold," flaxseed is one of the oldest known cultivated plants used not only for food, but also for making linen. It's a rich source of essential fatty acids, in particular omega-3's. As well as playing a critical role in normal physiology, essential fatty acids are shown to be therapeutic and protect against heart disease, cancer, autoimmune diseases such as multiple sclerosis and rheumatoid arthritis, many skin diseases, and other diseases. Numerous studies have uncovered the benefits of flaxseed to help alleviate constipation and bloating, eliminate toxic waste, strengthen the blood, reduce inflammation, accelerate fat loss and reduce depression.

Freshly ground flaxseed meal is extremely rich in omega-3's, dietary fiber, protein, mucilage and phenolic compounds. Sprinkle it on your salads, mix it in your smoothies, add it to your favorite recipes, or simply stir it into juice or water. The viscous nature of soluble fibers, such as flaxseed mucilage, is believed to slow down digestion and absorption of starch, resulting in lower levels of blood glucose, insulin and other endocrine responses. Grind your flaxseed meal fresh from organic golden flaxseeds (my favorite) and look for fresh sources of flaxseed oil in health food stores.

CONSIDER THIS: Within 1-3 days of adding flaxseeds to your diet, you will feel calmer. They have a positive effect on nervous energy. To help you eat less, 20-30 minutes before your largest meal of the day, drink a glass of water to which you've mixed in one tablespoon of freshly ground flaxseed.

11. GARLIC & ONIONS

A versatile culinary superfood with an ORAC score of 1,939, garlic has been around for ages. Herbalists and folk healers have used garlic to treat myriad diseases for thousands of years and it has been intensively studied in recent years with hundreds of scientific papers published in medical journals since the mid-1980's. The ancient Greek physician Dioscorides reported that garlic could "clear the arteries," and Hippocrates prescribed it for intestinal disorders. In 1858, Louis Pasteur discovered that garlic could kill bacteria. And because Russian physicians used the garlic bulb to cure infections, it was known as "Russian penicillin" well into the twentieth century. Albert Schweitzer is even said to have used garlic as a cure for amoebic dysentery when he was in Africa.

Not only healthy, garlic is scrumptious in many and varied food preparations; I always have several bulbs planted in my herb garden so I have fresh garlic greens to use. It's also a veritable treasure chest of nutrients. Garlic is a rich source of unique sulfur compounds that keep your body chemistry in balance. Similar to compounds found in onion, leeks, and chives, these sulfur compounds are thought to be responsible for garlic's antibacterial and antifungal activities, as well its ability to slow cholesterol synthesis, lower blood pressure, reduce atherosclerosis, and inhibit platelet aggregation.

The sulfur compounds in garlic may even prove helpful in fighting cancer. In the Iowa Women's Health Study, women who ate garlic at least once a week had a 32 percent lower risk of colon cancer than those who ate none. Research at the National Cancer Institute is showing that garlic extracts can both slow the proliferation of cancer cells and cause abnormal cells to self-destruct.

Further evidence points to garlic's cancer-fighting promise. Population studies have shown a decreased risk of colon cancer associated with consuming one to three servings (one to three cloves) of garlic per week. And it made no difference whether it was eaten raw or cooked. Cynthia Sass, M.A., R.D., a spokesperson for the American Dietetic Association, recommends that "anyone at risk for any cancer, including colon cancer, should include garlic as part of a plant-rich diet." Add the anticancer benefit to research showing that garlic may lower LDL (bad) cholesterol and kill harmful food-borne illness-causing bacteria and you have multiple reasons to enjoy garlic galore. It also adds flavor to your food without adding extra salt or calories. Many times monthly, my kitchen smells like roasted garlic and neighbors frequently comment on how they love the aromas coming from my kitchen windows.

The extract used in most garlic studies is called *Aged Garlic Extract,* also known as *Kyolic;* in fact, it has been proven effective in more than 460 studies—far more than all the other garlic products combined. That's because Aged Garlic Extract works for prevention and treatment of an amazing number of ailments— and it literally works wonders. I've perused all of the studies and have been so impressed that I've taken Kyolic Aged Garlic Extract for almost *40 years!*

Are you searching for a natural way to spark and strengthen your immune system? The medical community discovered Kyolic and the efficacy of its 12 to 14 month aging process which gives it the power to protect and enhance the health of our trillions of cells. Well-documented studies from major medical universities around the world have found Aged Garlic Extract to be effective in its ability to resist and fight cancer, cardiovascular disease, other respiratory ailments and infections, and fatigue. It also shows promise against homocysteine—a major risk factor in Alzheimer's disease and atherosclerosis. It's odorless and comes in a liquid extract, capsules and tablet form. For detailed information on Kyolic Aged Garlic Extract or for a free sample, visit: **www.kyolic.com** or call: **1-800-421-2998**.

> **CONSIDER THIS:** Instead of butter on whole grain bread, toast or crackers, I often use roasted garlic as the spread. I make large batches of it every couple weeks. You'll find myriad ways to use roasted garlic. The process of roasting softens the strong, pungent taste of raw garlic.

ONIONS. Whether green, red, white, yellow, or sweet, onions are members of the allium plant family, which also includes garlic, leeks, and shallots. Worldwide, the onion ranks number six as a vegetable crop; in the United States, it's number four. These versatile vegetables come in many sizes, colors, and flavors, and they are fat-, sodium-, and cholesterol-free and very low in calories. They add a taste sensation to any dish.

I admire onions for more than their flavor; their nutritional value is impressive, too. The green tops of spring onions are a good source of vitamin C and beta-carotene. Onions also contain quercetin, a potent antioxidant, and sulfur compounds which lower cholesterol. Recent studies give credence to the centuries-old belief about onions being a heart tonic. We now know that adenosine, a substance in onions, hinders clot formation, which may help prevent heart attacks. According to the book by Reader's Digest, *Foods that Harm, Foods that Heal,* onions may protect against the artery-clogging damage of cholesterol by raising the levels of protective high-density lipoproteins (HDLs). Still other studies suggest that eating ample amounts of onions may help prevent high blood pressure.

I'm sure you are familiar with one of the drawbacks of eating lots of onions: the result they have on your breath, which can even be detected on your skin. This pungency is caused by the sulfur compounds found in the onions. Perhaps you can overlook (or "oversmell") this drawback when you learn that onions also contain substances that have a mild antibacterial effect, which validates the old folk remedy of rubbing a raw onion on a cut to prevent infection.

Do you love onions but not like what happens to your eyes when you chop or dice them? The onions' sulfur compounds combine with enzymes to form a type of sulfuric acid, which is what brings tears to the eyes. On the bright side, this effect may help clear congested nasal passages during a cold. A syrup made from onions and honey is an old cough remedy. To cut down on the tears, try putting the onion in the freezer for 15–20 minutes before cutting it in addition to keeping your mouth open (breathe through your mouth, not your nose) while cutting.

> **CONSIDER THIS:** Shallots are a bit sweeter than onions and don't overpower a dish. I use them often in recipes.

12. KALE

One of the most nutritious greens in the garden, kale is part of the cruciferous family and is a rich source of indoles, glucosinolates and isothiocyanates, a group of potent phytochemicals that help prevent breast and lung cancers. The high content of the carotenoids lutein and zeaxanthin in kale helps prevent age-related macular degeneration of the eyes.

As a rich source of chlorophyll, kale oxygenates the blood, improves red blood cell counts and aids the fundamental processes of cell circulation and respiration. As if that wasn't enough, kale is also an outstanding source of beta carotene, vitamins C and E, and calcium. In fact, a cup of kale surpasses the calcium content found in a glass of milk and, because it contains an unusually high ratio of calcium to phosphorus, the calcium found in kale is absorbed far more successfully than that contained in dairy products. Adding to these accolades, kale is also rich in folate, iron, zinc, potassium and magnesium.

Few vegetables compare to kale when it comes to its nutritional beauty. The best way to feed your trillions of cells with this God-given treasure is by juicing it. Combine kale with other green vegetables and herbs (such as celery, Swiss chard, collard greens, romaine lettuce, cucumber, parsley, beet tops, etc.) and some carrot for sweetener. On an empty stomach, this super tonic will revitalize your cells and body in minutes.

> **CONSIDER THIS:** To make a delicious, nutritious green smoothie, blend 2 pears, 4-5 stalks of kale (with the tough center part cut out), and liquid of your choice until it's the right consistency for you. It will taste like pears but look green. I often sprinkle in some cinnamon before and after blending. I usually use water or fresh tea that I always have on hand and chilled.

13. KIWI

One of the most underrated of all fruits, the kiwi boasts a 602 ORAC score. This egg-shaped fruit with a fuzzy brown skin originated in China and was known as the Chinese gooseberry until New Zealand fruit growers renamed it for their national bird and began exporting it. Once considered an exotic fruit, kiwis are now grown in California and have become increasingly plentiful. They are harvested while green and can be kept in cold storage for 6 to 10 months, making them available for most of the year.

Kiwis are not only high in vitamin C, containing sixteen times more than oranges, but they also contain an impressive amount of vitamin E. The kiwi's bright green flesh, which is dotted with tiny edible black seeds, also provides a good amount of potassium as well as pectin, a soluble fiber that helps control blood cholesterol levels. A 3-ounce serving has only 56 calories and provides 85 mg of vitamin C. Kiwis also contain both lutein and zeaxanthin, antioxidants associated with eye health.

When shopping for this fruit, which has a somewhat tart flavor with overtones of berries, choose those with unbroken and unbruised skin. A ripe kiwi yields to gentle pressure. Most kiwis are sold hard and must be ripened at home. Ripen them at room temperature, out of the sun. Refrigerate ripe kiwis for up to one week. To enjoy, peel the skin with a sharp knife or a vegetable peeler. Slice crosswise. Kiwi will not discolor when exposed to the air and are a perfect choice for salads or garnish. Heating is not recommended, however, as the kiwi turns an unappetizing shade of olive green.

Once you discover the kiwi, it will grace your table often. I frequently add this luscious fruit to my morning smoothie for its rich array of vitamins, minerals, and phytonutrients in addition to its distinctive flavor. It's also a frequent companion to other fruit when I prepare a fresh fruit salad.

> **CONSIDER THIS:** Kiwis also come in a glorious gold-yellow color and brighten up any recipe. The esteemed kiwi is truly a feast for the eyes.

14. NUTS: ALMONDS & WALNUTS

What can be easier to snack on when you're hungry and on the go. Two ounces, or about 40 almonds, give you more than 50 percent of your daily requirement of magnesium, a mineral that's important for heart health. Almonds are also a good source of calcium, vitamin E, potassium, folate (the plant form of folic acid), fiber, and monosaturated fat, all heart-healthy nutrients.

In 2002, a study published in *Circulation* found that after eating about 2½ ounces of almonds a day for one month, participants had significantly reduced their total cholesterol and lowered several other risk factors for heart disease as well. Another study suggested that eating almonds may also reduce the risk of colon cancer.

One small extra step adds to nuts' nutritional value. Soaking nuts and seeds removes the growth inhibitors that impair germination, and once they germinate, seeds and nuts contain more life force and are easier to digest. During the germination process, each begins the transition from a nut or seed to vegetable.

After they've been soaked (they plump up and become softer) and then dried, keep almonds refrigerated. An alkalizing nut, almonds are great as part of trail mix, ground and mixed in a salad, used as part of a raw pie crust, or made into raw almond butter.

CONSIDER THIS: Almond milk can replace dairy milk in any recipe. Check out my almond milk recipe on page 233. With a few drops of vanilla and a sweetener of your choice, you'll have a versatile beverage to drink as is or use in smoothies or on top of whole grain cereal.

WALNUTS. A versatile and delicious nut, walnuts are the flagship nut because they alone provide two heart-healthy essential fatty acids: linolenic and linoleic fatty acids. Linolenic acid (an omega-3 fatty acid) is associated with a lower risk of coronary artery disease, according to a study published in the *American Journal of Clinical Nutrition* in 2001. Linoleic acid may reduce your chances of getting a stroke, according to a study published in *Stroke* in 2002.

Several clinical trials have found that eating walnuts lowers cholesterol. For example, in one study, men and women who ate about 2 ounces of walnuts daily for a month significantly lowered their total cholesterol. The plant sterols in walnuts play a significant role in lowering serum cholesterol levels. In another recent study, walnuts were found to keep a woman's heart healthy. In fact, walnuts recently were approved by the Food and Drug Administration for a qualified health claim stating that eating 1.5 ounces per day as part of a healthy diet may reduce the risk of heart disease. Studies also show that the omega-3 fatty acids found in walnuts may help prevent migraines. In the United States, 28 million people suffer from migraines, with women experiencing them more than men.

More reasons to appreciate this delicious raw food: walnuts are a good source of fiber and protein and they also provide magnesium, copper, folate and vitamin E. In terms of nuts, walnuts have the highest overall antioxidant activity. One of the main antioxidants is polyphenol, which may help prevent heart disease. Of course, nuts are also high in calories, but they have so many extraordinary health benefits and can be an important addition to your diet. Choose to eat a handful of nuts about five times a week. This simple act would reduce your chances of getting a heart attack by at least 15 percent and possibly as much as 51 percent, says Steven Pratt, M.D., in his book *SuperFoods.*

Dawn Jackson Blatner, R.D., L.D., a spokesperson for the American Dietetic Association, recommends using chopped walnuts in small amounts as a crunchy topping for low-cal foods like yogurt and oatmeal (walnuts are fairly high in calories—185 calories per ounce). Always select nuts that are fresh and raw, not roasted and/or salted. I also suggest eating them alone or incorporated in trail mix and sandwiches, chopped and sprinkled on salads and vegetables, added to whole grain cookies and breads and blended in smoothies and soups.

> **CONSIDER THIS:** Ten whole, raw walnuts (20 halves) one half hour before a meal helps keep a voracious appetite at bay.

15. PEPPERS: CHILIES & RED BELLS

A popular ingredient in Southwestern cooking, chilies—or hot peppers—add spice and interest to many foods. I consume the milder varieties as low-calorie, nutritious snacks. Have you ever noticed that you feel so good after eating chilies that you want more? According to Dharma Singh Khalsa, M.D., in his book *Food as Medicine,* that's because chilies raise your endorphin level. They're also a cornucopia of many nutrients, including impressive amounts of beta carotene and vitamin C. In fact, chilies are so rich in vitamin C that they have been used as natural remedies for colds, coughs, bronchitis and sinusitis around the globe. Just one raw, red hot pepper (1½ oz or 45 grams) contains about 65 mg of vitamin C, nearly 100 percent of the RDA.

Chili peppers are also chock-full of bioflavonoids, which are plant pigments that scientists believe help prevent cancer. Because chilies (red or green chilies and jalapeños) have been found effective in lowering low-density lipoprotein (LDL), they act as preventive medicine against strokes, high blood pressure, and heart attacks. Research also indicates that the ingredient that makes chilies hot—capsaicin—may help prevent blood clots that can lead to a heart attack or stroke by acting as an anticoagulant. Capsaicinoids, compounds found in chilies, have been incorporated into topical creams and recommended to help alleviate the pain of arthritis by simply rubbing it on aching joints.

Exercise some caution when handling chilies. When I'm preparing meals with chilies, I wear thin gloves, am careful not to rub my eyes, and always wash all utensils well with soap.

CONSIDER THIS: If you want to make a vegetable smoothie or juice spicier, include a teaspoon (or a few pieces) of some hot chilies, to taste, of course.

RED BELL PEPPERS. Another dieter's best friend, bells are the sweet peppers and, depending on their ripeness, they range in color from green to yellow to orange to red. Those picked while green will not become red, because peppers ripen only on the vine. Peppers grow sweeter as they ripen, which is the reason red ones are sweeter than yellow ones, which are sweeter than green ones. That's one of the reasons I prefer red bell peppers over the green ones. When green peppers ripen on the vine, they turn red and their vitamin content increases. So, like some people and wines, peppers just get better with age.

185

Peppers are a terrific, low-calorie, satisfying treat. A half-cup serving contains only 12 calories, but the vitamin content varies according to color. Ounce for ounce, peppers are a better source of vitamin C than citrus fruits. Because of this, I often eat them as a snack food, either cut into strips (great dipped in hummus) or I eat one whole as I would savor an apple. Just one serving of green peppers provides more than 100 percent of the adult RDA for vitamin C, whereas red peppers provide 50 percent more of this antioxidant. They are also a great source of beta-carotene, fiber, folate and vitamin B-6. Sweet red bell peppers come with an esteemed score of 710 on the ORAC scale.

A superb overall body alkalizer and healer, red bell peppers are an ideal ingredient that I juice or blend (mix them with other vegetables) in my healthy beverage recipes. These colorful veggies are a also breeze to roast; add the unique flavor of roasted red bell pepper to fresh hummus or other appetizing dips.

One word of caution, however, before you fill your grocery basket with these delightful gems. They are also on the top ten list of pesticide-laden vegetables when raised conventionally, so I highly suggest that you look for *organic* red, yellow, or orange bell peppers.

CONSIDER THIS: Cut the red (or any color) bell pepper in half for the perfect holder for finely chopped salads, dips, sauces, soups, etc. Don't forget to eat the bell after it's emptied.

16. POMEGRANATE

This dark red fruit is "hot" these days, especially in the form of pomegranate juice. Pomegranates boast disease-fighting antioxidants; some studies show that they offer almost three times the antioxidants of such well-known antioxidant super sources as green tea, red wine, blueberry juice, cranberry juice and orange juice. Not only that, pomegranates contain potassium, fiber, vitamin C, and niacin, which can all contribute to increased energy and good health. Research has shown that pomegranate juice reduced plaque buildup in arteries by 44 percent when given to subjects as reported in the *American Journal of Clinical Nutrition* 2000, 71:1062, which means it could also provide additional specific heart-healthy benefits.

Several scientific journals have published studies describing the promise of pomegranate. In *Atherosclerosis*, I read that "...pomegranate juice consumption can offer a wide protection against cardiovascular disease." From *The Journal of Nutrition,* "...pomegranate juice can contribute to the reduction of oxidative stress and atherogenesis." And from *The American Journal of Clinical Nutrition*, "Pomegranate juice treatment significantly and substantially inhibited the progression of atherosclerotic lesions (in mice)."

Jewel-toned red pomegranate juice is one of my all-time favorite beverages. I used to juice this fruit until I found the perfect source at my local farmers' market. So now, when pomegranates are in season and I mosey down to the farmers' market, I purchase two gallons of the freshly-squeezed, raw juice (you can also get the juice pasteurized and as part of fruit blends at your health food store). In addition to drinking this colorful elixir, I also make lots of frozen cubes from the juice to put in my water, in smoothies, and for use as part of the liquid base for chilled fruit soups. I also enjoy sucking on the frozen pomegranate cubes as a wonderful snack or dessert treat. Besides regular ice cube trays, I also have some in the shapes of hearts, fruit, flowers, teddy bears, and other animals. A heart of frozen pomegranate juice, or other fruit juice, is a lovely, special touch in a glass of water, tea or juice.

CONSIDER THIS: In a large glass pitcher, combine 2 cups of pomegranate juice, 2 cups of pure water, ⅓ cup fresh lime juice, and sweetener to taste. Stir and chill. Serve over ice for an exquisite, healthy drink or non-alcoholic beverage. Experiment with the best amounts of everything. It doesn't need to be exact; it also looks and tastes great.

17. SEA VEGETABLES: DULSE, KELP & NORI

Ounce for ounce, sea vegetables are a valuable treatment for candida albicans, as well as other immune-compromised diseases such as chronic fatigue, HIV infection, arthritis, and allergies. My three favorite sea vegetables—the ones I use most often in my diet and in my healthy food cooking classes and private culinary instruction—are dulse, kelp, and nori.

DULSE. An especially rich source of potassium, iron, iodine, vitamin B-6, riboflavin, and dietary fiber, dulse (*Palmaria palmata*) also provides a complete array of minerals, trace elements, enzymes, and phytochemicals, as well as some high-quality vegetable protein.

Incorporating dulse into my food program is as easy as a trip to my local health food store, where I buy this sea vegetable in granule form. It comes alone or mixed with garlic or other herbs and it's a great way to spice up your diet and detoxify at the same time. It is delicious sprinkled over spinach, popcorn, brown rice, and combined with walnuts. I also use it in soups, salads, dressing, dips, sauces, tabouli, potatoes, beans and more. It is a supremely balanced nutrient with 300 times more iodine and 50 times more iron than wheat. Research indicates it may fight the herpes virus. It has purifying and tonic effects on the body, yet its natural, balanced salts nourish as a mineral, without inducing thirst.

KELP. For a rich source of potassium, iron, iodine, riboflavin, dietary fiber, and vitamins A, B, C, E, D and K, kelp (*Laminaria*) has it all, plus is a natural substance that enhances flavor and tenderizes. Kelp contains sodium alginate (algin), an element that helps remove radioactive particles and heavy metals from the body. Algin, carrageenan, and agar are kelp gels that rejuvenate gastrointestinal health and aid digestion. Kelp works as a blood purifier, relieves arthritis stiffness and promotes adrenal, pituitary and thyroid health. Its natural iodine can normalize thyroid-related disorders like obesity and lymph system congestion. It is a demulcent (soothes and protects mucous membranes) and may help eliminate herpes outbreaks. Next time you want a seasoning, instead of salt, reach for kelp granules. I enjoy them plain and mixed with cayenne or garlic. A stellar, nutrient-dense sea vegetable, kelp can be found in health food stores.

NORI. This dusky-jade colored seaweed is more tender than other seaweeds. You're probably familiar with it as the flat sheet usually seen wrapped around a sushi roll. Like kelp and dulse, nori (*Porphyra tenera*) seaweed is a rich source of minerals and vitamins, especially vitamins A, B-1, and niacin. It has one of the highest protein contents of most seaweeds (48 percent of dry weight) and has been found beneficial in decreasing cholesterol, treating painful and difficult urination, edema, goiter, high blood pressure, and rickets; it aids in digestion, especially with fried foods.

You can purchase raw nori in sheets and eat it just "as is." I consume several sheets of raw nori weekly and often use it as a wrap for my salad ingredients. Build a wrap like a burrito by placing a handful of greens and other vegetables, such a grated carrots and beets, diced squash and tomatoes, and sliced onion and avocado, on the nori sheet. Drizzle on some dressing or hummus spread and wrap the nori around the veggies. You can also cut nori into strips with scissors, or crumble it over salads, dressings, and sauces. Try crisping it up by passing it over a low flame or baking it in a 300°F oven, just until the color changes. In this form, nori is typically added to soups and stews, or used as a condiment. When crisp, you can flake it by rubbing the nori between the palms of your hands; sprinkle these nutritious flakes on grains, salads, soups, etc.

CONSIDER THIS: Many of the skincare products that I use, by Reviva Labs, have seaweed as one of their main ingredients. Their *Hawaiian Seaweed Day Cream* stimulates, brightens, and softens the skin with energizing Hawaiian seaplant extract. *Reviva's Skin Energizing Gel* acts as a catalyst to stimulate skin cell energy; I use this gel before I moisturize. Additionally, I also love their *Seaweed Soap,* which I use as the perfect all-over body soap. Finally, I wouldn't be without *Reviva's Hawaiian Seaweed Beauty Mask;* for all skin types, this wonderful facial mask not only deep cleanses, it also moisturizes and brightens the skin. All of these products will help restore youthful vitality to your face and skin. For more information, or to purchase any of these stellar skincare products, please call: **1-800-257-7774** or visit: **www.revivalabs.com**. You will also find these products and all of Reviva's skincare line in better natural food and beauty stores.

18. SPICES: CINNAMON & GINGER

CINNAMON. Most people love the taste of cinnamon. Its fragrance conjures up thoughts of the holidays and special treats for the taste buds. An ancient spice obtained from the dried bark of two Asian evergreens, cinnamon is a highly versatile flavoring as well as a carminative that relieves bloating and gas. Adding cinnamon to food, especially to sugary ones, helps normalize blood sugar by making insulin more sensitive. Cinnamon's most active ingredient is methylhydroxy chalcone polymer (MHCP) which increases the processing of blood sugar by 2,000 percent, or twenty-fold. So using cinnamon in tiny amounts—even sprinkled in desserts—makes insulin more efficient. Cloves, tumeric and bay leaves also work, but they're weaker. This is great news! Avoiding high circulating levels of blood sugar and insulin may help ward off diabetes and obesity. Steady lower insulin levels are a sign of slower aging and greater longevity.

It's easy to get a "daily dose" of cinnamon. Most days I find ways to include cinnamon in my meals by sprinkling it on fruits and cereal, blending it in smoothies, and incorporating it in fruit sauces, purées, soups, and squash dishes. Don't forget to put cinnamon sticks in your tea or other hot beverage.

Here's one of my favorite breakfast or anytime-snack treats. I start with a generous amount of cut-up crisp romaine lettuce on a plate. Then I add large dice sections of pink or red grapefruit, orange sections and kiwi. And on top of it all, I sprinkle cinnamon. Absolutely delicious! Because of the high water content of the food, it's also very detoxifying and rejuvenating. Substitute any of your favorite fruits.

I also make sachets of cinnamon sticks, whole nutmeg and cloves—a thoughtful and easy-to-make gift. These sachets are wonderful hanging in the kitchen, closets, linen cupboard or laundry room.

CONSIDER THIS: In a diffuser, combine a couple drops each of cinnamon, lavender and vanilla essential oils (in some purified water) and let the fragrance take you to a peaceful, relaxed state of mind, even in the midst of a stressful day.

GINGER. The beige, knobby ginger root has a bite, a sweetness and a woodsy aroma all its own and is available year-round. Fresh ginger tastes decidedly different than powdered ginger. Cut off as much ginger as needed. Gently peel the thin beige skin from the root. The flesh beneath the skin is the most flavorful. Slice the ginger into "coins." Slices will lend an indirect flavor. Unpeeled ginger, tightly wrapped, can be kept in the refrigerator for about 3 weeks. I juice it, drink it as a tea, chop it for sautés and mince it for dips, sauces, soups and purées. Minced ginger will give a more pungent flavor. Look for robust roots with a spicy fragrance. Signs of cracking or withering indicate old age.

The centuries-old notion that ginger is health-promoting is now being confirmed by various types of research. Ginger contains several antioxidant plant chemicals, including gingerol, shogaol, and zingerone. These antioxidants help fight cancer and heart disease. Water spiked with ginger extract, when given to mice, significantly slowed the development of mammary tumors, according to a Japanese study published in 2002. Ginger extract lowered total cholesterol (and LDL cholesterol, too) and triglyceride levels and reduced atherosclerosis in mice as revealed in a 2000 Israeli study. And gingerol is as effective as aspirin in preventing blood clotting. It thins the blood "just like aspirin," making it a potential aid against heart disease.

In addition to being a powerful anti-inflammatory, ginger also promotes digestion and helps reduce or eliminate nausea (great for motion sickness and morning sickness). Anti-inflammatories are very important to overall health, since inflammation is a suspect in heart disease, stroke, cancer, Alzheimer's disease and arthritis. Gingerols reduce pain in animals and act as Cox-2 inhibitors, similar to the doctor-prescribed anti-arthritis drugs now available. University of Miami research shows that patients with osteoarthritis of the knee who took 255 milligrams of ginger extract twice a day for six weeks had less knee pain than those not getting ginger. So spice up your health and life with versatile gingerroot.

> **CONSIDER THIS:** I begin each morning with a large glass or two of purified, hot water to which I've added the fresh juice of ¼ to ½ lemon and 1-3 coins of ginger.

19. SPINACH

Popeye wasn't just a muscular cartoon figure; he knew what he was talking about when it came to his energy- and strength-building miracle food. This green goddess food is really one of the best body builders, cleansers, and rejuvenators you can eat.

One of my favorite leafy green vegetables (along with Romaine lettuce, arugula, and sunflower sprout greens), spinach is among the best sources of folate, which is critically important for cardiovascular and brain health. Low folic acid levels in your blood are associated with high levels of the amino acid homocysteine. Excessive homocysteine is a marker for increased risk of death resulting from heart disease. And since heart disease is a strong risk factor for memory loss, high levels of homocysteine are a marker for Alzheimer's disease as well. A half cup of boiled spinach contains 130 mcg of folate out of the 400 mcg you need to eat every day to keep your homocysteine levels under control. In a recent report, neurologists recommended eating spinach three times a week as a brain tonic.

Spinach also contains nearly twice as much iron as most other greens. Iron enables our red blood cells to carry more oxygen, which strengthens all cells but especially those of the brain and the respiratory system. About 15 percent of women of childbearing age are deficient in iron. Each half-cup serving of cooked spinach has over 3 mg of the 15 mg of iron you need daily. Fatigue is a symptom of iron deficiency. Lemon helps with absorption of this mineral which is one reason I generally sprinkle fresh lemon juice on my spinach. Moreover, because of its high iron content, spinach is a valuable food for the treatment of anemia, circulatory weaknesses, and cholesterol diseases such as hypertension and stroke.

Worried about your vision? Would you like to find an excellent food to support eye health? Look no further than versatile, scrumptious spinach. It contains an abundance of the two carotenoids mentioned previously, zeaxanthin and lutein, which help prevent age-related macular degeneration and retard the development of cataracts. Besides other green vegetables high in carotene, spinach plays a significant role against cancer. In one epidemiological study, women who consumed spinach regularly had a lower incidence of cervical cancer. Steven Pratt, M.D. in *SuperFoods* also selected spinach as one of the healthiest foods you can eat. It is one of the only two vegetables with a significant amount of coenzyme Q10; the other is broccoli. Coenzyme Q10 works in synergy with vitamins C, E, and glutathione. (Glutathione is the main antioxidant in cells. It is found in the watery interior of cells, where it protects DNA from oxidation.) Coenzyme Q10 is a key player in our skin's antioxidant defense mechanism against sunlight damage and also a significant player in mitochondrial energy production. (The mitochondria are the cells' energy factories.) Spinach is an important source of this critical antioxidant.

The minerals found in spinach are highly alkaline, which helps our bodies fight uric acid buildup and the symptoms of aging that go along with it. Another plus is that spinach is also high in oxalic acid, which interferes with calcium absorption. Raw spinach enables us to metabolize this acid better than the cooked variety.

When I visit my local farmers' market every week, I always buy a 3-pound box of organic baby leaf spinach. Then, throughout the week, I blend it for dips, soups, and vegetable smoothies, juice it with other vegetables, and eat it daily in salads. With all due respect to Popeye, lose the can! Instead, put a nice big handful of fresh, crisp, dark spinach leaves into your salad bowl or into your juicer. This chlorophyll-rich superfood is best when grown organically as spinach is also on the top ten list of pesticide-laden vegetables when raised conventionally.

CONSIDER THIS: Previously, I recommended blending pears and kale for a mouth-watering, nutritious green smoothie. Similarly, you can use a handful of spinach with pears, raspberries, mango, papaya, apples, etc., and the liquid of your choice for another green smoothie. I make one or more green smoothies every day. For more detailed information on green smoothies, including many delicious green smoothie recipes, please refer to my books *Health Bliss, The Healing Power of NatureFoods,* and *Recipes for Health Bliss.*

20. SUNFLOWER SEEDS & SPROUTS

One of my early mentors and friends in holistic medicine was the late Paavo Airola, Ph.D., author of many best-selling health books. Dr. Airola suggested that one of the staples of the human diet should be seeds and nuts, but always emphasized that we shouldn't overdo these foods because of their high fat content. A little bit goes a long way when it comes to seeds and nuts. According to Dr. Airola's research, all seeds and nuts should be eaten raw. One of his favorite seeds was the sunflower. They can be sprinkled on salads, made into sunflower seed butter or seed milk, made into delicious sprouts or ground into a meal.

Here's a simple recipe for basic sunflower seed milk that yields about 4 cups. Start with 1 cup raw, organic shelled sunflower seeds, 3 cups of pure water, and 1-2 tablespoons of your favorite sweetener like maple syrup, agave nectar or date sugar. Because sunflower seeds are so small, they don't require pre-soaking.

First, put the dry seeds in the blender and blend them to the consistency of nut meal. Now add in the water and continue blending. If you like your milk thick, do not strain the seed pulp when you're done. This gives your drink a rich milkshake consistency. Straining the blended seeds/water mixture will give you a lighter, smoother milk, if that's your preference. Sweeten to taste. You may also adjust the consistency by increasing or decreasing the amount of water. Use this scrumptious seed milk in any recipe that calls for milk.

Like most seeds and nuts, sunflower seeds are rich in vitamin E and potassium and high in minerals, including calcium, iron, magnesium and zinc. One ounce of sunflower seeds contains about 75 percent of the RDA for vitamin E. They are also rich in selenium, copper, fiber, folate and vitamin B-6. Sunflower seed butter makes a delicious high-protein salad dressing when diluted and blended with some lemon juice and purified water, fresh garlic, one tomato and your favorite herbs. It's also a great replacement for peanut butter on sandwiches and packed into the groove of celery. Make friends with these health-promoting seeds.

If you don't grow your own sunflower sprout greens from unhulled seeds, you can find them in the health food store. These sprouts are one of the best superfoods you can eat. I put them in smoothies, mix them in salads, and snack on them just as they are—delicious and nutritious. They usually can be found in the cooled vegetable section next to the other fresh sprouts.

CONSIDER THIS: Healthy trail mix makes a great, convenient snack. You can easily make your own with a combination of raw sunflower seeds, walnuts, almonds, and cashews mixed with raisins or goji berries. For a variation, add some shredded coconut and substitute dried cherries for the raisins and goji berries. You can't botch up the recipe. Just put in what looks good to you. Remember that raw nuts and seeds have more nutritional value than roasted ones.

21. APHANIZOMNENON FLOS-AQUAE (AFA)

For thousands of years, algae have been used worldwide as an excellent food source and potent medicine. For twenty-five years, the naturally occurring AFA growing in Oregon has been harvested and sold as a unique dietary supplement that's teeming with health-promoting compounds. "Although AFA grows in many other areas of the world," writes Christian Drapeau, MSc., in his book *Primordial Food Aphanizomenon flos-aquae: A Wild Blue-Green Alga with Unique Health Properties,* "the biomass that accumulates every year in Klamath Lake is unique in its abundance as well as its purity."

E3Live™ is 100 percent AFA. It's available in its complete fresh frozen liquid form. E3Live is collected only from the deepest, most primitive waters of Klamath Lake, Oregon, and harvested only at peak times of optimal growth, when the AFA is the heartiest, healthiest and most vibrant. For over twelve years, I've taken E3Live consistently, used it in my private practice, and highly recommend it to everyone. It provides more chlorophyll than wheatgrass; 60 percent high quality protein; all the B vitamins, including B-12; essential omega-3 and omega-6 fatty acids; and powerful digestive enzymes. It's also organic, kosher, vegan, raw and versatile.

E3Live is an abundant source of phycocyanin. Similar to chlorophyll, phycocyanin protects your body against toxins found in food, air and water. It also promotes healthy joint function and is an effective antioxidant. Similarly, E3Live is rich in PEA, a compound naturally produced by the brain that's released when we experience feelings of love, joy, pleasure and mental awareness. When taken orally, it is known to readily cross the blood-brain barrier and become immediately available to the brain. E3Live is the feel-good food—an excellent source of PEA.

World-renowned holistic physician/psychiatrist and author of several books, including *Conscious Eating,* Dr. Gabriel Cousens says this about E3Live: "As a physician working with thousands of clients, I find that E3Live helps to restore overall biochemical balance by nourishing the body at the cellular level. The positive response from the use of E3Live has been extraordinary. E3Live has the potential to enhance every aspect of our lives—mind, body and soul."

In my work with clients, I've seen E3Live help in the following ways: promote natural weight loss; reverse premature aging; increase strength and endurance; improve memory and concentration; stabilize mood swings; normalize cholesterol levels; promote strong nails, smooth skin and healthy hair; and provide deep sleep. Simply put: it gives you the full spectrum of over 64 perfectly balanced, naturally occurring vitamins, minerals, amino acids and essential fatty acids. E3Live provides immediate 97 percent nutrient absorption, nourishing the body at the cellular level and helping to restore overall biological balance.

CONSIDER THIS: Commit to taking E3Live for 90 days and see how great you feel. To order, visit: **www.E3Live.com** or call: **1-888-800-7070, 1-541-273-2212**.

So there you have it. See how many of these 21 superfoods you can include in your diet to prevent disease and create youthful vitality and vibrant health.

> FOOD IS A LOVE NOTE *from God.*
>
> — GABRIEL COUSENS, M.D.

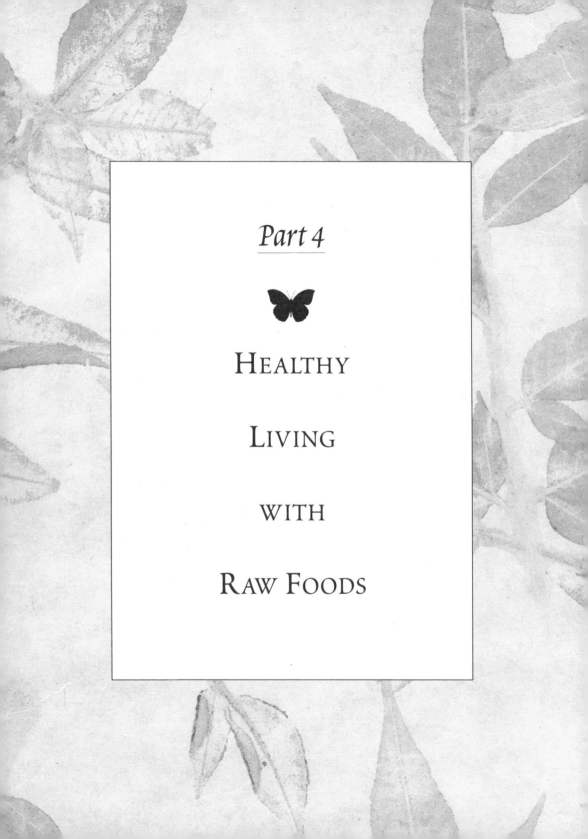

Part 4

HEALTHY

LIVING

WITH

RAW FOODS

REJUVENATE WITH 40 LIFE-AFFIRMING RECIPES

Each cell of the body is like a tiny battery, and raw and living foods supply the bio-electricity which charges these batteries.

— RHIO

In Part 4 I provide 40 delicious, easy-to-prepare recipes that I have created to assist you in gently and expeditiously rejuvenating your body, mind, and spirit. Experiment with each one and see how you can make them different and equally scrumptious. You will soon notice that none of these recipes require heat. They are all nutrient- and enzyme-rich and support the overall health of the body and mind.

I encourage you to eat as much raw food as possible. Consider taking two days each week—perhaps Monday and Thursday—and make those your living food days. On the other days, eat at least 60 percent of your diet raw. For more information on easy recipes and specific foods that heal your body and promote radiant health, please refer to my books, *The Healing Power of NatureFoods, Health Bliss,* and *Recipes for Health Bliss.*

Many of the recipes require a blender, which I write about in "Create a Healthy Kitchen," Part 2, number 12, of this book. Invest in the best one that you can afford. With a top-quality blender, you'll become a gourmet cook and you can create wonderful, rejuvenating smoothies, soups, sauces, dips, nut and seed butters, tonics, elixirs, and nutritious blends in literally seconds. Blender snacks or meals are very easy to digest, because the machine has done much of the work for you, thus making these treats very detoxifying and rejuvenating on your body.

The same goes for a juicer. Buy a top-quality, multi-purpose juicer such as the *Champion;* it's an indispensable machine in a healthy kitchen. (See page 96 for some recommendations.)

Few of us have time to spare in the kitchen even though we strive for better health. I appreciate healthy meals and treats that take less than 15 minutes to prepare. That's what you'll find here: special rejuvenating treats to bolster your health, promote vitality, and rejuvenate your life. The following recipes are all nutrient-rich and restorative to the body.

> IN THE TYPICAL WESTERN LIFESTYLE, *we get in the way of our own health by congesting our cells and ourselves with processed and hard-to-digest food. Live food infuses one's being with fresh, vibrant energy, helping us feel invigorated and revitalizing our capability to resist disease.*
>
> — BRIGITTE MARS

COOL COCONUT–FRUIT SMOOTHIE 1

This is one of my favorite smoothies that I have a few times each week. It's nutrient-rich and takes only a couple minutes to make. Vary the fruits from blueberries, raspberries, or blackberries to peaches, cherries, papaya, mango, banana, or kiwi, separately or a combination of two or more. With each different fruit, it boasts a new, glorious color and a variety of nutrients. I usually use just one fruit so I can enjoy the rich color and sensational taste of the fruit.

- **2 to 3 young coconuts**
- **2 cups frozen fruit**

  (Serves 2 to 4)

You can find young coconuts at natural food stores or better grocery stores. If you can't find them, ask the produce manager to get you a case of them. Cut off the top of the coconut with a sharp knife. Pour the coconut water into a blender. Scrape out the coconut meat with a spoon and add this to the mixture. Next, add the frozen fruit and blend until smooth using extra coconut water or purified water to reach your desired consistency. Pour into glasses and serve.

2

SIMPLE & STRONG
CLEANSER/REJUVENATION TONIC

First thing in the morning, as an afternoon pick-me-up, or to use throughout the day as a one- to three-day rejuvenating cleanse, this simple-to-make tonic will incite your cells to sizzle with enthusiasm and vitality. I've been drinking this for over three decades and recommend it often to friends and clients. This is my signature tonic that I created 30 years ago as an alternative to Stanley Burroughs's The Master Cleanser. Studies reveal that the chemical composition of the coconut water and coconut meat is only a few molecules different from your blood's plasma. I have a glass of pure coconut water mixed with some fresh lemon juice several times a week to help foster vibrant health and youthful vitality.

- **2 cups water from young chilled coconuts**
- **1 tablespoon fresh lemon juice**
- **⅛ teaspoon organic cayenne pepper**

(Serves 2)

Stir and serve.

VARIATIONS: You can substitute 1 cup fresh pineapple or apple juice for 1 cup of water. Coconut water is the best, however, and the most healing and rejuvenating.

SCRUMPTIOUS NON-DAIRY "CHEEZE"

3

For those of you who aren't familiar with cheeze, this is my name for a nondairy source of cheese. Different kinds of nuts and seeds create different flavors of cheeze. Cashew cheeze tastes like Philadelphia cream cheese. Almond cheeze (skins removed) tastes like ricotta. Sunflower cheeze has a sweet taste, but it's gray in color. The process is the same for all these delicious, versatile cheezes.

- **4 cups cashews, soaked in filtered water for about 12 hours and drained**
- **1 to 1½ cups Rejuvelac**

(Makes about 4 cups)

Blend the Rejuvelac and cashews. Use just enough liquid to barely cover the nuts or seeds. When the mixture is smooth (20–30 seconds), pour it into a sprout bag (or cheese cloth) and hang overnight. The whey (liquid part) will drain out and separate from the curds (solid part). The cheeze should smell slightly sour and cultured, like yogurt. Drain as desired for a firmer cheeze and save the whey to use again. You can shape, pack, and store the cheeze in a bowl or container for a desired shape, and refrigerate it for up to 3 days.

VARIATIONS: Almond cheeze is my favorite, especially when I've taken time to remove the skins after they've been soaked. You can also make colorful, festive cheeze rolls, dips, and spreads by adding avocado, minced garlic, parsley, basil, cilantro, chopped onion, bell peppers, carrots, juice and zest of lemon or lime; pinch of nutritional yeast; hydrated, chopped sun-dried tomatoes, onion powder; pesto with flax, etc.

Flavor the cheeze with your favorite sweetener and blend with fresh fruit to make a sensational torte, pie filling, or frozen dessert.

4
REJUVELAC
(FERMENTED GRAIN BEVERAGE)

Rejuvelac is a high acidolphilus culture-grain drink made popular by Dr. Ann Wigmore, a visionary woman who brought sprouts and wheatgrass to the world. This beverage provides vitamins, minerals and an impressive supply of healthy bacteria and enzymes helpful in the digestion process. Drinking this salubrious tonic improves the alkaline balance and strengthens the immune system. Start with small quantities of Rejuvelac so that your body can become accustomed to its cleansing properties. Six to eight ounces a day, working up to a quart a day, is adequate for most people. I use Rejuvelac as a base for smoothies, shakes, soups, dips, sauces, cheezes, etc.

Here's my favorite way to make Rejuvelac that I learned from raw food cuisine educator Cherie Soria. If you want to make it wheat-free, you can substitute the grain, kamut, for the wheat berries.

- **¼ cup soft wheat berries**
- **¼ cup whole rye**
- **2 gallons purified water**
- **Fruit-flavored tea bags are optional to enhance the flavor.**

(Makes 2 quarts each day for 3 days)

Day #1: In the morning, combine the grains in a gallon jar (preferably glass), cover with plastic mesh, and secure with a rubber band. Add at least 2 quarts of water and soak 8–12 hours. That evening, pour off soak water, rinse with tap water, and drain well. Place jar in a cool, dark place and allow to sprout.

Day #2: In the morning, rinse and drain again, and repeat this process in the evening.

Day #3: In the morning, rinse once with tap water and drain well. Rinse again with purified water, drain, and add 2 quarts purified water. Put jar in a cool, dark place and ferment 36–48 hours. (It will ferment sooner in hot weather.)

Day #5: In the morning, pour your first batch of fermented water (Rejuvelac) into a container and store in the refrigerator to drink that day. Pour 2 more quarts of purified water onto the sprouted grains (do not rinse!) and allow to ferment another 24 hours.

Day #6: In the morning, repeat step #5.

Day #7: The final morning, pour your third batch into a container and store in the refrigerator to drink that day. (To stretch your harvest for a fourth day, repeat step #5.) Discard grains and wash jar well with soap and water.

VARIATIONS: In my experience, the first batch is the strongest. Simply add a fruit tea bag to the Rejuvelac after it has been fermented to enhance the taste, if you wish.

FYI: To have Rejuvelac all week long, I start new batches two times every week. You must use filtered, not chlorinated water, or it won't work. Chlorine kills the bacteria and friendly flora. It takes 5 days from the time you soak the grains to when you have Rejuvelac to drink. If you have been on the Standard American Diet (SAD), because Rejuvelac is so cleansing, you might want to start with smaller amounts, as mentioned above. I usually drink a quart a day and am always using the liquid to make special cheezes and scrumptious recipes.

5   SUMMER BREEZE FRUIT SMOOTHIE

Rich in enzymes, antioxidants and phytonutrients, low in calories, and a superb alkalizer and rejuvenator, papaya is a superfood indeed. The unripe fruit contains a milky juice that has a protein-digesting enzyme known as "papain," which greatly resembles the animal enzyme pepsin in its digestive action. This juice is used in the preparation of various remedies for indigestion.

- **2 ripe bananas, peeled**
- **1 mango, peeled, seeded and cubed**
- **1 papaya, peeled, seeded and cubed**
- **1 cup fresh pineapple chunks**
- **Ice cubes to taste**

(Serves 2 to 3)

Blend until smooth and serve. If you want a gift to your taste buds with something really special, add the water and soft meat from a young coconut.

RUBY GRAPEFRUIT & STRAWBERRY SMOOTHIE

6

Strawberries, blueberries and raspberries are naturally low in fat, a good source of fiber, and rich in vitamin C. Red grapefruit is a great source of beta carotene and lycopene. Deep inside the white rind and membranes of this fruit (lemons and oranges, too) lies a miraculous group of plant compounds—bioflavonoids, citric acids, and pectins. These plant compounds protect against cancer and heart disease.

- **2 cups ruby red grapefruit juice**
- **1 cup strawberries, frozen**
- **2 teaspoons coconut butter**

  (Serves 2 to 3)

Blend and serve in a glass with a strawberry slice on the glass rim.

TIP: I Prefer to use only unheated coconut butter.

7   # HEALTH-BOOST APPLE COOLER

Coconut butter contains no cholesterol and does not elevate bad (LDL) cholesterol levels. The medium-chain fatty acids (MCFA's) in coconut butter possess incredible properties that are a natural antibacterial, antiviral, and antifungal. Just make sure you get a good source that's unheated, and if possible, hand-crafted and organic. You can usually find this in a natural food store.

- **2 apples, peeled, seeded and quartered**
- **2 tablespoons coconut butter**
- **1 cup apple or pineapple juice**
- **½ cup almond milk**
- **1½ cup ice cubes**

(Serves 2 to 3)

Blend and serve.

SAVORY PERSIMMON-FIG SHAKE 8

Whether using fuyu, hachiya, or cinnamon persimmons, these gems of nature will add pizzazz—as well as a treasure trove of nutrients— to any recipe. This colorful shake will dress up any elegant dinner party as easily as it will be enjoyed by everyone at your next picnic or tailgate party. For those of you who like your fruit shakes thick and cold, add 3-4 ice cubes before blending.

- **1 to 2 ripe persimmons**
- **¼ cup pumpkin seeds, soaked for 4 hours and drained**
- **2 dried figs, soaked for 1 hour**
- **⅔ cup fig soaking water**
- **1 banana**
- **⅛ teaspoon cinnamon**
- **⅛ teaspoon cardamom**

(Serves 1 to 2)

Blend and serve.

9   WATERMELON & SUPER-BERRY SMOOTHIE

By itself, watermelon eaten all day long, without consuming anything else, is a wonderful detoxifier and rejuvenator once a month or with each change of season. It's over 95 percent water, takes stress off the digestive system, and is a rich source of lycopene. Strawberries are very high in vitamin C, potassium, and antioxidants.

- **2 cups watermelon, seeded and diced**
- **1 cup frozen raspberries, or strawberries and blueberries**
- **1 tablespoon lemonade concentrate**
- **½ cup ice cubes**

(Serves 2 to 3)

Blend and serve.

AUTUMN APPLE-APRICOT BLEND

10

Next time you're feeling a bit peckish, try this satisfying smoothie.

- 4 apricots, pitted
- 1 cup apple juice
- 1 apple, quartered and cored
- 1 banana, peeled
- 5 to 6 frozen cubes of almond milk
- 1 tablespoon sweetener (optional)

(Serves 2 to 3)

Blend and serve.

TIP: Try making the first batch without additional sweetener— I prefer it that way.

11   SPICE-IT-UP TOMATO JUICE

Over 90 percent of this beautiful, low-calorie fruit, the tomato, is water. It's alkaline and jam-packed with nutrients and phytochemicals, including lycopene. The best tomatoes are home-grown or purchased at local farmers' markets. They are available in all colors from red to gold, orange, green, and yellow. And because most of the nutritional value is contained in the skin, ounce for ounce, cherry tomatoes afford more nutritional value than large tomatoes, although I use large tomatoes for this recipe.

- **2 cups ripe tomatoes, quartered**
- **¼ cup chopped bell pepper green, red, or yellow,**
- **¼ cup chopped onion**
- **⅛ teaspoon garlic powder or fresh minced garlic**
- **¼ teaspoon sweetener**

(Serves 1 to 2)

Blend to desired consistency and serve.

TIP: I prefer red or yellow bell peppers but green's okay if you like. Add sweetener only if necessary.

WONDERFUL WATERMELON REFRESHER

12

When you add deep reds or bright pinks to your daily diet, you are adding a powerful antioxidant called lycopene. Lycopene is found in tomatoes, red and pink grapefruit, watermelon, papaya and guava. Diets rich in lycopene are being studied for their ability to fight heart disease and some cancers. Lycopene also can raise the sun protection factor (SPF) of the skin. In other words, it acts like an internal sunblock.

- **4 cups watermelon, diced**
- **½ cup strawberries, frozen**
- **1 tablespoon frozen limeade concentrate**

(Serves 1 to 2)

Blend for a few seconds and serve in chilled glasses with a sprig of mint on the top.

13   MARVELOUS MELON MIX

Melons provide a wealth of vitamins A, B, and C, along with trace minerals and enzymes. On a hot summer day, everyone loves this beautiful, delectable smoothie.

- **2 cups watermelon chunks**
- **2 cups honeydew melon chunks**
- **½ cup cantaloupe chunks, frozen**
- **½ cup strawberries, frozen**
- **1 tablespoon pure maple syrup or agave nectar (optional)**

(Serves 2 to 3)

Blend and serve.

VARIATIONS: Substitute frozen pitted cherries or blueberries for the strawberries.

POWERHOUSE BLEND ELIXIR **14**

If you find yourself getting teary-eyed over onions, try one of these remedies: 1) Freeze the onion for half an hour before chopping; 2) Peel onions under running water; 3) Don't slice the onion root, which releases the strongest fumes.

- 1½ carrots
- ¼ beet
- 1 tablespoon fresh parsley
- 1 stalk celery cut in eight pieces
- ½ cucumber, peeled
- 1 tablespoon onion
- 1 apple, cored and quartered
- 1 cup apple or carrot juice (to sweeten)
- Ice (optional)

(Serves 2 to 3)

Blend to desired consistency and serve.

15   ZINGY LEMON/FRUIT COOLER

Bananas are a good source of vitamin C, potassium and dietary fiber. The banana plant is not actually a tree; it's the world's largest herb. Although acid to the taste, the juice of a lemon is a great alkalizer for the body. When our bodies are too acid, our immune systems are compromised and our energy abates. Of all the citrus fruits, lemon is the most potent detoxifier. Studies also reveal that adding zest from citrus fruit (lemons, grapefruit and oranges) to food may help prevent skin cancer. Strive for at least one tablespoon of fresh zest each week.

- ½ cup cold water
- 1½ cups strawberries, fresh or thawed
- 2 cups peach slices, frozen
- 1 ripe banana, peeled
- 1 can frozen lemonade (6 ounce)
- 1 tablespoon lemon zest

(Serves 2 to 4)

Blend to desired consistency and serve.

LUCKY PEACH SMOOTHIE

16

In China, the peach is a symbol of longevity and good luck!

- ¼ cup fresh coconut butter
- 1 cup fresh peaches, pitted
- ⅓ cup almond milk
- 1 cup ice cubes

(Serves 1 to 2)

Blend and serve.

17 CHERRY SUPREME SHAKE

This blend is as beautiful to look at as it is delicious to drink. Enjoy it any time of the day.

- 1½ cups almond milk
- ½ cup apple juice
- 1 cup cherries, pitted, fresh or frozen
- ½ cup blueberries, fresh or frozen
- 2 medium bananas
- ½ cup raw cashews
- ½ vanilla bean

(Serves 2 to 3)

Blend until smooth.

VARIATIONS: If you want it colder and more like a shake, use frozen fruit or add some ice cubes.

CLASSIC STRAWBERRY-BANANA SMOOTHIE

18

The combination of high vitamin C strawberries and high potassium banana is a nutritional winner and the beautiful rose color of this smoothie also nourishes the soul.

- **8 frozen strawberries**
- **1 ripe frozen banana, cut into chunks**
- **⅔ cup fresh strawberry juice (if you don't have a juicer, substitute apple or orange)**
- **½ cup vanilla yogurt or soy yogurt**
- **2 tablespoons frozen apple juice concentrate, thawed**

(Serves 2 to 3)

Blend and serve.

VARIATIONS: If you don't have a juicer, substitute apple or orange juice for the strawberry juice. To increase protein, add 1 to 2 scoops of your favorite protein powder.

19   RAINBOW BERRY DELIGHT

Blue and purple fruits not only add beautiful shades of tranquility and richness to your plate, they add health-enhancing flavonoids, phytochemicals, and antioxidants. Blueberries, in particular, are rich in vitamin C, folic acid and potassium, and are also high in fiber.

- 1¾ cups apple juice
- ⅓ cup blueberries, frozen
- ⅓ cup strawberries, frozen
- ⅓ cup raspberries, frozen
- ⅓ cup blackberries, frozen
- ¼ cup raw cashews
- ½ cup ice

(Serves 3 to 4)

Blend to desired consistency and serve.

PASSIONATE POMEGRANATE SMOOTHIE

20

The pulp (seed) of the pomegranate fruit is 82 percent water and contains 63 calories per 100 grams of the edible portion. One pomegranate provides most of the body's daily potassium and vitamin C needs, a healthy dose of fiber, and no fat. Next to pure water and the water from a young coconut, fresh pomegranate juice is one of my favorite, healthy beverages that I have several times a week. Make ice cubes from the pomegranate juice for flavoring water or tea, or blending into smoothies.

- **1½ cups pomegranate juice**
- **½ cup blueberries, frozen**
- **½ cup strawberries, raspberries, or blackberries or a combination, frozen**
- **1 banana, peeled**
- **Ice**

(Serves 2 to 3)

Blend to desired consistency and serve.

TIP: Pomegranate juice is available at natural food stores and local farmers' markets. If I don't juice it myself, I purchase unheated juice.)

21 | MAGICAL CINNAMON-PEAR SMOOTHIE

Adding cinnamon to food, especially to sugary ones, helps normalize blood sugar by making insulin more sensitive. Cinnamon's most active ingredient is methylhydroxy chalcone polymer (MHCP) which increases the processing of blood sugar by 2,000 percent, or twenty-fold. So using cinnamon in tiny amounts—even sprinkled in desserts—makes insulin more efficient. Cloves, turmeric and bay leaves also work, but they're weaker.

- 1½ cups pears, peeled, cut into chunks and frozen
- 1 ripe frozen banana, cut into chunks
- ¾ cup almond milk
- 2 ounces of raw cashews
- ⅛ to ¼ teaspoon cinnamon

(Serves 1 to 2)

Blend until smooth.

SUPER VITALITY PROTEIN SHAKE

22

I make this smoothie, or a variation, several mornings a week right after my workout. It really hits the spot and provides a balance of high protein, healthy carbs, and omega-3 fatty acids.

- 2 to 3 cups liquid—use Rejuvelac, fresh juice, hemp milk, water, tea (like organic green tea), or nut milk made from almonds or cashews (see page 233 for the recipe)
- 1 ripe banana, peeled
- 1 cup fresh or frozen fruit such as blueberries, strawberries, raspberries, blackberries, cherries, papaya, peaches
- 3 to 4 leaves of romaine lettuce
- 1 ounce raw walnuts, almonds or both
- 1 tablespoon flaxseed
- 1 tablespoon Living Harvest Hemp Protein Powder
- 1 tablespoon salba seeds (rich in omega-3s, fiber, protein, etc.)

(Serves 2 to 3)

Blend, adding extra liquid, if necessary. Serve immediately.

VARIATIONS: For the liquid base, I frequently use some Rejuvelac along with a tea mixture. Sometimes I add fresh ginger, vanilla or cinnamon powder. I might also incorporate a few raw pumpkin seeds or sunflower seeds. To make it really creamy, try adding a handful of raw cashews instead of the walnuts and almonds. If you want it colder and more like a shake—especially if you are using fresh fruit rather than frozen fruit—blend in a few ice cubes.

TIP: Living Harvest Protein Powder available at: **www.livingharvest.com**

23 | APPLE-PLUM SUPER SMOOTHIE

"Dried plums" is really another way of saying prunes, which sometimes get a bad rap. This is a refreshing, potassium-rich afternoon pick-me-up guaranteed to keep you in the flow.

- **1 cup almond milk**
- **8 prunes, pitted**
- **½ cup frozen apple juice concentrate**
- **¼ lemon, peeled (outer layer only, keep pithy part on)**
- **⅛ teaspoon ground cinnamon**
- **3 leaves of fresh mint**
- **5 to 6 ice cubes**

(Serves 1 to 2)

Blend until smooth and serve.

PURE & SIMPLE ALMOND MILK

24

Almonds are a great source of protein and are very alkaline. They are the king of nuts, providing calcium, magnesium, phosphorus, potassium, zinc, folate, and vitamin E. Fresh almond butter is heavenly. Cashews provide calcium, magnesium, iron, zinc, and folate. Protein-rich sunflower seeds are best eaten raw and unsalted and can be sprinkled on salads, made into sunflower seed butter, sprouted into rejuvenative green sprouts, or ground into a meal and used in pie crusts. Let's not forget the beautiful sunflower plant that brightens any home or garden.

- **1 cup raw almonds**
- **6 cups purified water**

(Makes about 5 cups)

Soak the raw almonds in 2 cups of water for at least 6 hours (the first step in sprouting). In a blender, add the presoaked and drained almonds with 4 cups of water. Blend on high until creamy. If you prefer it more like the consistency of dairy milk, strain it through a fine strainer or cheese cloth to remove fiber. This keeps 3-4 days in the refrigerator. Chill and serve.

VARIATIONS: To sweeten, add pure maple syrup, agave nectar or a few pitted dates and blend, or add raw carob powder and you have "chocolate milk." I also like it with a sprinkle of cinnamon powder. You also can substitute sunflower seeds or cashews for the almonds but you don't need to soak either of them.

TIP: Nuts change from about 25 percent protein and 75 percent fat to about 75 percent protein and 25 percent fat when sprouted.

25 COCO-NANA-DATE SHAKE

From toddlers to seniors, I have never found anyone who does not love this shake. No matter the season, it is always a favorite and it is actually good for you. I sometimes have this healthy shake for a meal or afternoon snack. Coconut contains some phytosterols that are cholesterol lowering. It is also a good source of soluble fiber, known to lower cholesterol.

- **2½ cups almond milk**
- **2 small or 1 large ripe frozen banana**
- **5 to 6 medjool dates, pitted and chopped**
- **2 tablespoons unsweetened, shredded coconut (or fresh meat, if you have it)**
- **4 to 5 ice cubes**

(Serves 2 to 3)

Place all the ingredients in a blender and blend until creamy smooth. Add more or less almond milk for desired consistency.

VARIATIONS: Adding some vanilla extract brings a special flavor to this shake. To increase the vitamins, minerals and antioxidants, I often add some frozen fruits such as blueberries, raspberries, blackberries, mango, papaya, peach. If you want to make a Chocolate-Date-Peppermint Shake, to the above recipe, add 2 tablespoons pure organic cocoa powder (or raw carob powder) and ⅛ teaspoon peppermint extract. Carob has enjoyed increased popularity in recent years as a low-fat, low-calorie, low-caffeine alternative to chocolate.

MORE VARIATIONS: If you want it colder and more like a shake, use frozen fruit or add some ice cubes. Carob has enjoyed increased popularity in recent years as a low-fat, low-calorie, low-caffeine alternative to chocolate.

COOL-OFF CANTALOUPE SOUP WITH LIME

26

This raw and refreshing soup is perfect on a hot summer day! It's teeming with antioxidants, beta-carotene, potassium and vitamin C.

- **2 ripe cantaloupe, cut into chunks**
- **1 cup fresh orange or tangerine juice**
- **⅓ cup fresh lime juice**
- **1 teaspoon grated fresh ginger root**
- **½ organic lime, thinly sliced**
- **4 to 6 fresh mint sprigs**

(Serves 3 to 6)

In a blender, puree the melon, orange juice, lime juice, and ginger. Pour into serving bowls and chill in the bowl. Garnish each serving with a slice of lime and a sprig of mint.

VARIATIONS: Substitute honeydew melon or apricots for cantaloupe and fresh apple, peach, nectarine, or strawberry juice for the orange juice.

27 LIVE-IT-UP TOMATO-VEGGIE SOUP

This nutrient-rich soup takes only a few minutes to make and is a perfect fast food. It's replete with antioxidants, enzymes, lycopene, vitamin C, selenium, and beta-carotene. If you want to lose some weight, have a cup as your first course before lunch or dinner. It fills you with nutrients and volume so you will not eat as much afterwards. I also put this soup in a thermos or bottle and take it with me when I'm out all day or traveling. It's great hot, warm or chilled. Vary the vegetables (tomatoes are really a fruit) according to what you have available. It is so easy, healthy, fast and a delectable raw food meal or snack.

- 1 cup liquid, hot (water, tea, broth, fresh veggie juice, etc.)
- 5 large or 6 medium tomatoes cut in half
- 1 cup purple cabbage, cut in chunks
- 1 cup baby carrots, peeled
- ¼ to ½ small onion, peeled
- ¼ cup fresh basil leaves (optional)
- 1 to 3 cloves garlic (optional)
- Mint and basil leaves for garnish

(Serves 2 to 4)

Blend until smooth and serve in heated bowls if you prefer it warm or hot. Garnish with sprigs of mint and/or basil.

VARIATIONS: Some other vegetables and herbs I frequently add include parsnips, yellow squash, celery, parsley, basil, arugula, spinach, green onions, jalapeño peppers, string beans, zucchini, and cucumbers. For added seasoning, try unpasteurized miso.

VERSATILE VEGGIE
SMOOTHIE-OR-SOUP

28

Here is a great way to "eat" your vegetables! The combination of miso and mint may sound odd but they add a wonderful balance of flavors to this veggie drink.

- **2 cups fresh carrot juice**
- **1 cucumber, peeled if not organic**
- **1 bell pepper, red, yellow or orange**
- **6 leaves romaine lettuce**
- **3 leaves cabbage, green or purple**
- **1 cup spinach**
- **½ cup fresh sunflower seed sprouts**
- **½ small lemon, with peel if organic**
- **½ avocado, pitted and peeled**
- **¼ cup raw cashews**
- **½ to 1 tablespoon organic miso**
- **2 to 3 teaspoons flaxseed**
- **Mint sprigs, for garnish**

(Serves 3 to 4)

Juice enough carrots to make 2 cups. Continue to juice the other produce (cucumber, pepper, lettuce, cabbage, spinach and lemon). Pour mixture into a blender and add avocado, cashews, flaxseed, and miso. Blend until smooth and serve in chilled glasses with a sprig of mint, or warm in a mug on a cold day.

VARIATIONS: You can use any vegetables or veggie juice you have on hand. If you do not have a juicer, then simply blend all of the ingredients until smooth, adding extra liquid until you reach your desired consistency. For liquid, you can use almond milk, green tea or other teas, purified water or vegetable broth.

TIP: Try tossing in a clove of garlic or 1 teaspoon of KYOLIC (aged garlic extract: **www.kyloic.com**)

29 YOUNGER-EVERY-DAY COCKTAIL

This free-radical scavenger cocktail will do wonders for boosting immunity and restoring youthful vitality.

- **1 cup organic green tea, freshly brewed and chilled**
- **4 medium carrots, washed but not peeled**
- **1 red or green apple, cored and quartered**
- **½ cup broccoli sprouts**
- **1 stalk broccoli, including florets**
- **½ cup cauliflower**
- **3 leaves romaine lettuce**
- **¼ red bell pepper**
- **¼ yellow or orange bell pepper**
- **¼ wedge lemon with peeling, if organic**
- **¼-piece fresh ginger root**

(Serves 2 to 3)

Juice everything and serve with a lemon wedge.

NATURAL BEAUTY BLEND 30

Drink this daily for a week. Your skin will glow, your eyes will sparkle, and your energy will soar.

- **1 medium red or green apple**
- **1 red, yellow, or orange bell pepper**
- **3 medium carrots**
- **3 leaves romaine lettuce**
- **2 stalks celery**
- **½ medium cucumber**
- **¼ wedge lemon with peeling, if organic**
- **¼- to ½-inch piece fresh ginger root (optional)**

(Serves 2)

Juice all the ingredients together, and serve.

31   SIMPLE SLEEPYTIME SIPPER

Taken an hour before bedtime, this delicious combination is guaranteed to help you fall asleep without having to count sheep.

- **1 cup freshly brewed chamomile tea**
- **2 apples, cored and quartered**
- **2 stalks celery**
- **¼ cup parsley**

(Serves 1 to 2)

Juice the apples, celery, and parsley, then mix with the tea. Sip slowly.

SERENITY SIPPER

32

If you're feeling irritable or anxious, this colorful drink will lift your spirits and lower your stress levels. Lemon balm is an herb and member of the mint family. It is reported to help combat mild forms of anxiety and irritability. (Pregnant women and people with hypothyroidism should not use lemon balm.)

- **1 ruby red grapefruit, outer skin peeled (leave pithy part on)**
- **1 pear**
- **8 strawberries, with green tops**
- **1 cup freshly brewed lemon balm tea**
- **¼-inch piece fresh ginger root (optional)**

(Serves 2)

Juice all the fruits (and ginger, if using) and mix with the tea. As you drink this tonic, make sure to breathe slowly and deeply.

33 CANCER-BUSTING VIBRANT V-12

After tasting this delicious vegetable juice, you'll never want to drink the canned varieties again.

- 4 large ripe tomatoes
- 3 large carrots
- 3 stalks of celery
- 1 bell pepper, yellow, red, or orange
- 4 green onions
- 4 leaves of the greenest romaine lettuce
- 4 large leaves of spinach
- 2 leaves of kale
- ½ cup of broccoli sprouts
- ½ small beet
- ⅓ cup parsley
- 1 to 3 cloves garlic
- 1 small lemon with peeling, if organic
- ¼ teaspoon living Celtic Sea Salt

(Serves 2 to 3)

Juice all the ingredients. Add extra tomatoes at the end if you need more juice. Stir in the salt.

TIP: You can find Celtic Sea Salt online at **www.celtic-seasalt.com**. I order many health products from this company monthly, including the *Selina Naturals* line of products.

TANGY ENERGY TONIC 34

This spicy drink stimulates circulation and helps rev up metabolism by creating heat and energy. I usually double or triple this batch and keep it on hand. Pour some into ice trays and freeze, using the frozen cubes in water or tea. If you're familiar with Yogi tea or chai, this is like a minty version of these popular Indian teas.

- 3 cups purified water
- 4 slices (¼-inch) fresh ginger root
- 4 cinnamon sticks, cut in half
- 1 tablespoon dried peppermint, either loose or in a tea bag
- ½ teaspoon cardamom seeds
- ⅛ teaspoon whole cloves

(Serves 2)

In a medium saucepan, combine all the ingredients and simmer for about 10 minutes. Strain and drink hot or cold.

35   READY-SET-GO MORNING ELIXIR

If you don't have much time for breakfast but want a healthy start to the day, this vegetable and fruit combination fits the bill. I've enjoyed this drink several times each week for three decades.

- **3 medium carrots**
- **1 apple**
- **1 large stalk celery**
- **1 stalk broccoli, with florets**
- **⅓ cup parsley**
- **¼ sweet bell pepper (orange, red, or yellow)**
- **½ small beet, scrubbed**
- **¼ lemon wedge with peeling, if organic**
- **¼-inch piece of ginger**

(Serves 1 to 2)

Juice all ingredients, and serve.

VARIATIONS: If I want something more substantial, I'll put this juice in a blender and add 1–2 tomatoes, one cup of sunflower seed sprouts, about 10 soaked almonds, 2 tablespoons of golden flaxseeds, and ½ cup cucumber. For extra protein, I might add some organic hemp powder from *Living Harvest.* Blend and serve. It's also great in the afternoon for a pick-me-up beverage or blender meal. I usually make a double batch so I can have some throughout the day as needed.

POWERHOUSE SALSA SUPREME 36

Besides using salsa as a dip for baked chips and raw vegetables or a variety of Mexican dishes, you might want to use salsa on everything from brown rice, millet, or quinoa, as a topping on baked potatoes or steamed vegetables, or wrapped in lettuce leaves or nori (sea vegetable) sheets with some avocado slices, grated carrots, and other vegetables.

- 1½ cups tomatoes, diced
- 2 tablespoons finely diced white onion
- 1 tablespoon red bell pepper, finely diced
- 1 tablespoon yellow bell pepper, finely diced
- 1 to 2 tablespoons fresh cilantro, chopped
- 2 teaspoons fresh lime juice
- 1 jalapeño chili, seeds and white rib removed, minced
- 1 teaspoon minced or pressed garlic
- ⅛ teaspoon minced ginger
- Sea salt to taste (I use ½ teaspoon of Celtic Sea Salt. Add just before eating.)

(Makes about 2 cups)

Combine all the ingredients thoroughly in a bowl. Refrigerate until ready to serve.

VARIATIONS: For Corn Salsa, add ½ cup corn kernels cut right off the cob. For Mango Salsa, add ½ cup diced mango. For Avocado Salsa, add ½ to ¾ cup diced avocado.

TIP: Most of the chili's heat is in the white tissue (the ribs), not the seeds as most people think. If you want a hotter salsa, leave in the white tissue and seeds and mince the whole thing. I recommend wearing gloves when you do this and keeping your fingers out of your eyes.

37 APPLE-SALSA DELIGHT

When you want a quick, nutritious snack or side dish or if you're in the mood for some Tex Mex flavor, try this colorful dish. It's high in antioxidants and is a great source of fiber and omega-3 fatty acids.

- **3 large or 4 medium red delicious apples, cored and chopped**

- **1 cup salsa**

- **3 tablespoons raw walnuts, chopped or ground**

- **2 tablespoons freshly ground flaxseed**

(Serves 3 to 4)

Wash, core, and chop the apples and put in a bowl. Mix in the remaining ingredients. Serve immediately or chill. I always make it fresh and add the salsa at the last minute, right before serving.

VARIATIONS: Dice the apples into smaller pieces and use this recipe as a dip for fresh vegetables, baked chips, or as a sandwich spread in pita or on whole grain bread.

TIP: I prefer to use golden flaxseed.

AMAZING AVOCADO BOATS WITH SALSA

38

It can't get much simpler than this. Ounce for ounce, avocados provide more heart-healthy monosaturated fat, vitamin E, folate (the plant source of folic acid), potassium and fiber than other fruit. Yes, it is a fruit! I eat this as a snack or with meals as a salad. Vegetables from the onion family, which include garlic, chives, scallions, leeks, and any variety of onion, contain the phytochemical allicin which may help lower cholesterol and blood pressure and increase the body's ability to fight infections.

- **1 unpeeled avocado, halved lengthwise and pitted**
- **4 tablespoons salsa**
- **1 tablespoon chives, chopped**
- **Fresh greens**

(Serves 2)

Put ½ avocado on a bed of lettuce greens and fill the hole with the salsa and chives. Enjoy every delicious bite of avocado, known as nature's butter, topped with salsa and chives.

39   SUPER VITALITY SALAD

You can't get much tastier than this simple, crispy salad. A great rejuvenator and mild cleanser, this salad lends itself to any favorite occasion.

- 2 cups romaine lettuce, torn into small pieces
- 1 cup baby leaf spinach, torn or left whole, stemmed
- 1 cup arugula

THEN ADD:

- ½ cup chopped celery
- ½ cup shredded carrot
- ½ cup shredded beet
- ½ cup diced jicama
- ½ cup diced ripe tomato
- ½ cup diced cucumber
- ¼ cup diced bell pepper, red, yellow, or orange
- ¼ cup sunflower seed sprouts
- ¼ cup broccoli sprouts
- Edible organic colorful flowers, for garnish

(Serves 3 to 6)

In a bowl, combine all ingredients and toss with your favorite dressing.

VARIATIONS: To add more protein to your salad, add some beans such as garbanzo beans or black beans, edamame (out of the pods), sunflower or pumpkin seeds, grilled tofu slices, or perhaps a scoop of quinoa or millet, to make this a perfect complete meal in a bowl.

OPTIONS: Following are two salad dressing options to liven things up.

This easy, healthy, and delicious vinaigrette is my favorite dressing that I've used more than any other for years. To get the most juice from a lemon, roll it back and forth on a hard counter for a few seconds, then cut it, and squeeze. Some books and chefs tell you to microwave it for a few seconds to make it juicier, but I don't recommend this method because cooking destroy all of the enzymes.

SUPER VITALITY VINAIGRETTE

- ⅓ **cup fresh lemon juice**
- 2 **tablespoons organic balsamic vinegar**
- ⅓ **cup fresh, organic flaxseed oil**
- 1 **teaspoon garlic, pressed**
- 1 **teaspoon Dijon mustard (optional)**
- ⅛ **teaspoon Celtic Sea Salt**

(Makes about ¾ cup)

Whisk together the lemon juice, vinegar, garlic, mustard, and sea salt until well blended. Drizzle in a little oil at a time, whisking after each addition until all the oil is thoroughly incorporated. Use within 3 days.

VARIATIONS: You can substitute other vinegars, such as raw apple cider vinegar, raspberry, brown rice, red wine, etc., either for half or all the balsamic vinegar.

SUPER VITALITY FRENCH VINAIGRETTE

- ¾ **cup basic Vitality Vinaigrette**
- 1 **large ripe tomato, cut into quarters**

(Makes 2 cups)

Blend on high for 15 seconds. Use within 3 days.

VARIATIONS: Add 1 to 2 teaspoons of any of the following chopped or minced fresh herbs: basil, chervil, chives, thyme, cilantro, dill, Herbes de Provence, lemon grass, mint, oregano, parsley, rosemary, tarragon.

40   MULTI-BERRY MIRACLE SORBET

Here's a refreshing and fruity treat that will have you smiling from ear to ear with the first spoonful. The flavors and texture will cleanse the palate or put an exclamation point after any meal.

- **1 frozen banana**
- **⅓ cup frozen raspberries**
- **⅓ cup frozen blueberries**
- **2 tablespoons cherry concentrate**
- **2 teaspoons lemon zest**
- **2 cubes of frozen almond milk**

(Serves 2)

Blend and serve.

VERY VANILLA COCONUT PUDDING · 41

From children to seniors to those with the most discriminating palates, here's a delightful, delicious treat that brings generous smiles and requests for seconds.

- **Meat of 3 young coconuts**
- **1 cup medjool dates, soaked for 20 minutes and drained**
- **1 teaspoon vanilla extract or 1½- to 2-inch vanilla bean**
- **¾ cup coconut water**
- **Cinnamon (optional)**

(Serves 3 to 4)

Purée all ingredients in a food processor and serve the pudding in cups. Sprinkle some cinnamon on top.

VARIATIONS: This is the basic recipe. To increase the nutritional value, add a panoply of color, and a wow! taste sensation, I often add berries, such as blueberries, strawberries, raspberries, and blackberries. I also enjoy it with a blend of other fruits such as banana, mango, papaya, cherries, peaches, nectarines, pears, plums, prunes, tangerines, oranges, or kiwi. Try adding some fresh citrus zest such as lemon and orange or some fresh, minced ginger. Garnish the top of the pudding cup with the same fruit that you added to the purée. Savor every bite.

For more delicious, nutritious, and easy-to-prepare recipes and revitalizing foods that heal your body, promote radiant health, and rejuvenate your life, please refer to my 3-book *Hay House Healthy Eating & Living* series—*The Healing Power of NatureFoods, Health Bliss,* and *Recipes for Health Bliss.*

NEVER BE DISCOURAGED *by your progress. You're changing deeply rooted, lifelong habits—ones that may be life threatening but have become a very real part of life for you—into new ones that may be lifesaving; that takes time!*

— CAROL ALT

SUSAN'S FAVORITE HEALTH PRODUCTS

*When you are loving yourself by taking good care of yourself
and living a balanced life, you are loving God.*
—SUSAN SMITH JONES

Since I receive more than 1,000 letters each year asking for a list of my favorite health products, I thought I would take this opportunity to mention a few of them here. Throughout every nook and cranny of this book, you will find other health-promoting products (and their contact information) that have made a positive difference in my life. Be perspicacious and check all of these products out. If you visit my website and click on *Susan's Favorite Products,* you'll find that I discuss some of them in more detail. I even have a variety of radio interviews that you can listen to for more information.

ACTIVATED AIR BY ENG3

A remarkable health machine that I wouldn't be without, Eng3's Activated Air devices help the body's cells use oxygen better. Since oxygen and nutrients from food are the only sources of fuel for the body, activated air—like good nutrition—can make a big difference to your health. An Activated Air device is about the size of a small printer. Normal air is altered inside activation chambers of the device, so that your cells can more easily utilize the oxygen in the air. A single user, through a nasal cannula, then inhales the activated air. Typically the device is used 20 minutes to an hour, three to seven times a week. It is cleared as an Inhalation Device by the FDA and is registered as a Class I Medical Device.

Activated Air is used to protect against oxidative stress by triggering the oxidative response system. Oxidative stress is the result of excessive free radical accumulation from aging, over-exertion, toxins in your food or environment, and other lifestyle factors. Some of the more common disorders associated with oxidative stress include the following: Asthma and other respira-tory illnesses, cancers, cardiovascular diseases, chronic fatigue, diabetes, fibromyalgia, macular degeneration, neurological dis-orders, pulmonary diseases, a range of mitochondrial diseases, and many other disorders. To determine if a specific disease is associated with oxidative stress, you can search the Internet with the name of the disease and the term "oxidative stress." If the disorder you are concerned about is related to oxidative stress, Activated Air may be the answer for you because it triggers the body's oxidative response system to protect against, and repair, the damage of oxidative stress. The outcomes include, but are not limited to:

- Protection against free radical damage
- Repair of damage already caused by free radicals
- Improved oxygen utilization
- Improved cell energy production
- Improved cell metabolism

Even if you are more proactive, like I am, and are not addressing a specific disorder, Activated Air will still help improve your health. As we age, our cells' ability to effectively use the oxygen in the air we breathe drops dramatically, even when we practice deep breathing on a regular basis. Activated Air will optimize your oxygen supply and make a positive difference in how you feel. This superlative device was developed by European scientists to combat this drop in efficiency and to help us keep our cellular energy production in top shape. Maximizing the cell's ability to produce energy (ATP) is the best protection against illness and the effects of aging. Simply put: optimized cellular energy production improves our overall health and quality of life; retards age-related diseases and disorders; reduces damage from excess free radicals; enhances cellular regeneration; maximizes our ability to draw nutrition from the food we eat; improves athletic performance; and shortens recovery time. While Oxygen therapy such as that found in Oxygen bars will give you a boost in energy, it has no long-term positive effect on your health. Activated Air, on the other hand, improves your body's ability to use the oxygen you're already breathing and cuts down on free radical pollution that—doctors say—causes a variety of diseases and even aging itself. A plethora of scientific studies speak for themselves and, because our space is limited here, I encourage you to check these out for yourself.

I've seen noticeable, positive differences in how I look and feel and how my clients feel after using it. On a personal note, because of Activated Air, I now sleep better, have an easier time concentrating and focusing on my work, exercise harder without tiring, recover more rapidly, and have more energy than I ever dreamed possible, among a long list of other noticeable benefits. If you are interested in losing weight, definitely consider purchasing an Activated Air. Oxygen is the key to burning fat. With maximized oxygen uptake, you can use fat more easily as your body's fuel source. In other words, you'll probably have an easier time losing weight—you may experience an acceleration of fat loss, especially when combined with an optimum diet (described in this book) and regular exercise. I've seen this over and over with my clients.

Activated Air is completely natural and contains no chemicals or drugs of any kind; it's the best way I know to help make oxygen more available to your cells. Completely safe, it can be combined with other treatments. It can be used in the privacy of your own home or office. I even take it with me when I travel. Refer to my website and click on *Susan's Favorite Products,* for a write-up on Activated Air and why I recommend it to everyone. For more detailed information or to order, please visit: **www.eng3corp.com** or call: **1-877-571-9206.**

AGE IN REVERSE

Larry Jacobs, the founder and owner of this renowned company, has created the most wonderful anti-gravity products that I've used and recommended for decades. For more information or to order, please visit: **www.ageeasy.com** or call: **1-888-Age-Easy.**

ALKALIFE

AlkaLife drops boost the pH value of any drinking water, changing it into healthy alkaline water. The recommended dosage is 4 drops in a 6- to 10-ounce glass of water and drinking 5 glasses a day. AlkaLife can also be taken with tea, coffee, or juice, but not with carbonated drinks or dairy beverages. The 1.25-ounce bottle of AlkaLife contains approximately 1,200 drops and will last you about two months, consuming 20 drops a day. I carry the small bottle with me everywhere I go, especially when I am traveling. For more information or to order, please visit: **www.alkalife.com** or call: **1-888-261-0870.**

ANCIENT SECRETS NASAL CLEANSING POT

The practice of nasal irrigation, known as Neti, has been used by practioners of Yoga and Ayurveda in India for thousands of years. Some yogic teachers consider it valuable in cleansing the energy channels and balancing the right and left hemispheres to create radiant, energetic health and wellness. Many people practice Neti on a daily basis to keep their sinuses clean and improve their ability to breathe freely. Most find it a soothing and pleasant practice once they try it.

If you are one of the many people who find that your nasal passages are blocked as a result of the effects of pollution, dust, pollen and other irritants, you may find this simple cleansing technique of invaluable benefit to you. While there are advanced techniques using various herbs and herbal oils, the simplest technique, and the one I practice often, uses water for the cleansing process. Lukewarm water is used to gently open up the nasal passages.

Doctors and alternative health practioners around the world recommend the regular practice of nasal cleansing using a saline solution (I mix sea salt with warm water) as part of a regular regimen of health and well-being. While the practice of nasal irrigation may have originated in India, today there are large numbers of people in Europe and North America who have added this simple technique to their daily hygiene.

Not only have I been doing nasal irrigation for over 30 years,

I also highly recommend it in my private practice; I especially recommend it for anyone with sinus problems and environmental allergies. Within 30 days of practicing neti, one to two times a day, I've seen many clients and friends no longer need allergy medications after a lifetime of use. Some of the other many benefits of using the Nasal Cleansing Pot include the following: clears the nostrils to free the breathing; removes excess mucus; reduces pollen or allergens in the nasal passages; relieves nasal dryness.

While many companies offer nasal cleansing pots, the only one that I use and recommend, because it's the best, is the Ancient Secrets® Nasal Cleansing Pot by Lotus Brands, Inc. Their pot is crafted from sturdy, lead-free ceramic (not plastic) and coated with food-grade sealant glaze; it's a heavy-duty construction that's diswasher safe. It makes nasal irrigation easy and enjoyable. I've included more information on nasal cleansing on my website; simply click on Susan's Favorite Products. To order my favorite Nasal Cleansing Pot by Ancient Secrets, please visit: **www.ancient-secrets.com/neti.cfm** or call: **1-877-263-9456.**

BERNARD JENSEN INTERNATIONAL

You'll notice that I recommended the books, *Tissue Cleansing Through Bowel Management,* by Dr. Bernard Jensen, and *Health is Your Birthright* by Ellen Tart-Jensen. Everyone should read these books if you're interested in being your healthiest and keeping your body detoxified and rejuvenated. It's impossible to look and feel your best if you do not have a healthy bowel system. For 35 years, I have been a proponent of dry skin brushing, which I write about in detail in my book, *Health Bliss*. Briefly, the practice of dry skin brushing helps detoxify the body, cleanse the colon, and improve circulation. Along with daily dry skin brushing, you'll want to undertake a dynamic detoxification program to help balance your internal environment, at least four times a year. With each change of season, I undertake a cleansing program, and I also do a monthly three-day cleanse. For all of my monthly and quarterly cleanses, I use and recommend the *Internal Cleanse Tool Kit #1* or *#2* by Ellen Tart-Jensen. This kit contains everything you need to totally cleanse and rejuvenate right down to a cellular level. When I am doing a personal cleanse program, I also take extra capsules of *Super Organic Rainbow Salad*. For more information on all of these products or to order a dry skin brush, the Internal Cleanse Tool Kit or Super Organic Rainbow Salad capsules, please visit: **www.bernardjensen.org** or call: **1-888-743-1790** (outside the United States—**1-760-471-9977**).

CHAMPION JUICER

For over thirty-five years, I've used and recommended the *Champion Juicer.* Designed with simplicity in mind, the Champion doesn't require nuts, bolts, screws or clamps. Assembly can be completed in seconds; cleaning is equally quick and easy. This machine is designed to produce the highest quality fruit and vegetable juices and foods. It's a difference you can see in the color of the fresh juice: darker, richer colors contain more of the pigments—and nutrients—you desire, while the extracted pulp is pale in color. And rest assured, it's a difference you can taste. In my Champion, I make everything from leafy greens and vegetable juice, fruit juice, and melon and citrus juice, to fruit sauces and purees, sorbets, sherbets, and ice cream (from fresh, frozen fruit), to dessert toppings, baby foods, and nut butters, to freshly ground flour, corn or soy meal, and ground spices. The juicer comes in a variety of colors. For more information, please refer to my website, click on Susan's Favorite Products, and listen to my radio interview discussing the Champion Juicer. To order, please visit: **www.championjuicer.com** or call: **1-800-WE JUICE (935-8423)**

E3LIVE

This is one of nature's most perfect superfoods, and the world's first and only fresh-frozen live *Aphanizomenon flos-aquae* (AFA). For thousands of years, algae have been used worldwide as an excellent food source and potent medicine. For 25 years, the naturally occurring AFA growing in Klamath Lake, Oregon, has been harvested and sold as a unique dietary supplement that's extremely nutrient rich. AFA provides more chlorophyll than wheatgrass; it's 60 percent high qaulity protein; it has all the

B vitamins, including B-12; it provides essential omega-3 and omega-6 fatty acids; and it is teeming with powerful digestive enzymes. It is the only AFA product that is organic, kosher, vegan, raw and so versatile.

For over twelve years, it's been a staple in my diet and a healthful food I recommend to everyone. It is a delicious green liquid that lends itself to combining with water, adding to juices or smoothies or simply enjoying it by the tablespoon. I encourage you to try it for ninety days—just one season—and see all of the positive beneifts it will have on your physical, mental, emotional and spiritual well-being. You'll find information on E3Live on my website when you click on *Susan's Favorite Products.* Ask the company, *Vision,* the harvesters of E3Live, to send you their excellent free CD that describes the product beautifully and what it can do for your hair, skin, body, and overall well-being. For more detailed information or to order, please visit: **www.e3live.com** or call: **1-888-800-7070.**

EXCALIBUR FOOD DEHYDRATOR

These paramount dryers have changed the way health conscious people all over the world view food preparation and enzyme preservation. From drying fresh fruit, to creating gourmet raw foods, these dryers may soon replace the microwave oven in the health-savvy home. For more information or to order, please refer to my website, click on *Susan's Favorite Products,* and read my article, *Fun & Easy Food Dehydration,* or listen to the radio interview. Please visit: **www.excaliburdehydrator.com** or call: **1-800-875-4254**.

HERBAL ANSWERS

Their aloe vera juice and topical skin gel have been part of my health program for years; I wouldn't be without either. Their products are the best of their kind available, carefully created to retain and protect the potency, integrity and biological activity of the entire fresh aloe plant as originally designed by Nature. You can order these products through the company or through The Grain & Salt Society (see below). For more information on these must-have products, visit: **www.herbalanswers.com** or call: **1-800-256-3367**.

HYDRO FLOSS

How you care for your teeth and gums has a direct impact on your overall health. That's why I use my Hydro Floss oral irrigator daily. To learn more about the efficacy of this appliance or to order one, visit: **www. oralcaretech.com** or call: **1-800-635-3594**.

IONIZER PLUS

As we alkalinize our bodies, we maximize our health. This advanced ionizer first filters the tap water to remove contaminants, chlorine, chemicals, taste, and so forth. Next, it enters an electrolysis chamber which divides it into Alkali-ion and Acidic-ion water. The reduced molecular clusters permeate the body quickly and efficiently. The *Ionizer Plus* is paramount in my health program. I use the alkaline water for drinking and for meal preparation and the acid water for my skin and plants; I wouldn't be without mine. For more information, visit my website and click on *Susan's Favorite Products*. To order, please visit: **www.hightechhealth.com** or call: **1-800-794-5355.**

MAXGXL

Here is a glutathione supplement (a stellar antioxidant) that I wouldn't be without in my personal holistic health program. I also highly recommend it to all of my family, friends, and clients. I have seen it reduce or eradicate many "dis-eases" that result from eating the Standard American Diet (SAD) and living out-of-balance lives. MaxGXL has made a profound difference in my life—from how I look and feel, to my energy level, to how much better I sleep and focus.

Briefly, this is why I believe everyone should include this supplement in his or her diet. The human body was designed by God to be self-healing and to maintain optimal health. It was designed to receive the nutrients to sustain vibrant health from a diet consisting of primarily raw, colorful plant-based foods free of chemicals and toxins. Unfortunately, in the day in which we live, it is often difficult to achieve and maintain an optimal level of wellness even with the best of diet and lifestyle. The foods of today lack much of the nutrition that the same foods contained just a few decades ago. We live in an environment where not only many of our foods are toxic from chemicals and environmental pollution, but our water and air are also polluted. It has become increasingly more important to supplement our diet with nutrients that support radiant health and youthful vitality.

One of the most important elements of health is glutathione, the master antioxidant in the body. As we age, due to the environmental conditions we live in, our body's ability to produce glutathione decreases from 10 to 12 percent per decade after the age of twenty years. Supplements of glutathione are useless since they are degraded in the stomach environment. Up until recently, the only effective way to increase the body's glutathione levels was by intravenous injections. To see some of the many benefits of intravenous glutathione and its impact on disease, please visit: **www.glutathioneexperts.com/gsh-diseases.html.**

Fortunately, because of a remarkable discovery resulting from ten years of research by Robert Keller, MD, today we now have the ability to facilitate our body's production of glutathione at cellular level by as much as 300 percent. Dr. Keller's research provides us with a supplement containing the necessary precursors for the body's natural production of glutathione. Regarding Dr. Keller's research, Dr. John Nelson, the 159th president of the American Medical Association has this to say:

> This product, in my opinion, represents the single most important breakthrough in health that I will witness in my lifetime. I believe it will revolutionize, change, and transform the practice of medicine worldwide and make Dr. Robert Keller more famous than Jonas Salk—who created the polio vaccine.

Now you can take advantage of Dr. Keller's remarkable research and take this superlative glutathione accelerator each and every day, as I do, and also get wholesale pricing as a Preferred Customer by ordering through the following website: **www.4HealthBliss.com**, and click on Preferred Customer or call **1-801-316-6380.** You will thank your lucky stars that you found out about this breakthrough supplement and are making it part of your daily health regimen. I wouldn't be without it.

REVIVA SKIN CARE PRODUCTS

One of the most-asked questions I receive, whether participating in media talk shows, giving workshops, or consulting with clients, goes something like this: "Susan, what skin products do you use? Your skin looks so healthy and youthful!" I usually respond by saying that healthy skin starts on the inside and results from eating a top-quality diet (as described in this book) and drinking plenty of water each day. Of course, you must also get enough sleep, keep stress to a minimum, protect your skin from excessive sun exposure, exercise regularly, do a dry-skin brush daily, and cultivate a positive attitude.

But—it's also important to use good skin care products. For over thirty years, most of the products that I've used on my skin have been made by the eminent company *Reviva Labs*. Established in 1973, Reviva realized long before there was an emphasis on "natural" that natural ingredients were essential in order to have healthy skin. While Reviva offers a complete line of superb products for all skin types, some of my favorites include their *Light Skin Peel, Green Papaya Hydrogen Peroxide Facial Mask, Optimum Antioxidant Facial Mask with Artichoke,* and all of their seaweed-based products.

I use the Light Skin Peel once a week on my face and neck and on the back of my hands. A non-chemical peel, this celebrated mask/peel helps improve color tone, refine and smooth skin texture, and brighten skin surface. The beautiful feel and look of your skin after removing the peel is a result of its ingredients—papaya extract, salicylic acid, almond and root extracts, zinc oxide, and kaolin—that, combined, dissolve dead skin and leave you with a very healthy glow.

Then, usually right after the peel, but sometimes on an alternate day, I might follow up with the Hawaiian Seaweed Face Mask, the Green Papaya Hydrogen Peroxide Facial Mask or the Optimum Antioxidant Facial Mask with Artichoke. Beyond cleansing pores of impurities and pollutants, these masks deliver fresh ingredients that will help your skin look clearer and more radiant. Because of the natural ingredients, your skin will benefit without redness or irritation. These are soothing, soft, non-hardening, non-drying masks that can benefit any skin type, even sensitive skin like mine; they will leave your skin sparkling clean, smooth and glowing. I use these masks on my face, neck, décolleté, and the backs of my hands.

You can find these products, and most of the Reviva product line, at better natural food or beauty stores. For more detailed information or to order direct from the company, please visit their website: **www.revivalabs.com** or call: **1-800-257-7774.**

THE GRAIN & SALT SOCIETY

This top-quality company is where I purchase my Celtic Sea Salt and many other healthy products on a regular basis. They carry only the best-of-the-best products and they ship anywhere in the world. I encourage you to call and request a free sample of their superb Celtic Sea Salt as well as their catalog and their newsletter, *A Grain of Salt*. My articles are often featured in their informative, motivating newsletter. For more information or to purchase any of their numerous and varied beneficial products, please visit: **www.celticseasalt.com** or call: **1-800-867-7258.**

THE TOTAL BLENDER AND KITCHEN MILL

Indispensable in my healthy kitchen, cuisine classes, and private culinary instruction, the blender is a miracle to me. I use mine several times every day to make soups, smoothies, vegetarian "cheese" sauces, dressings, nut milks, "ice cream," purees, and nut butters. The grand prix of all blenders is made by Blendtec®. Called *The Total Blender*™, the price is higher than the regular department store blenders—and it's well worth it! This machine has no problem chopping ice or blending nuts and seeds into delicious butters. Less expensive machines are great for smoothies, soups, and dressings, but you will have to be careful not to burn out the motor when making nut cheeses or nut butters. Before I discovered this blender, I burned out a few other blenders.

Blendtec also makes a superlative grinding mill that can transform dry wheat, rice, corn, oats, rye, beans, peas, and other legumes into fresh flour in seconds. This efficacious *Kitchen Mill*™ grinds with low heat, so the nutrients and enzymes are saved. When you mill your own flour with the push of a button— and keep all the nutrients intact—you can put together the most nutritious, delicious meals. Like the blender, this mill is a must-have tool to assist you in preparing salubrious complex-carbohydrate, protein, and whole-grain meals that will fortify your body and optimize your health. For more information or to order The Total Blender or the Kitchen Mill, visit my website and click on *Susan's Favorite Products*. You'll also find a radio interview where I discuss "Blending Made Easy." For more information, please visit: **www.blendtec.com** or call **1-800-253-6383.**

EVERYDAY HEALTH—
PURE AND SIMPLE

Sure-Fire Tips to Heal Your Body, Restore Youthful Vitality & Renew Your Life—Audio Program by Susan Smith Jones

In this encouraging, heartwarming interview, Dr. Susan Smith Jones provides all the tools you need to walk away from the darkness of doubt and confusion, and into the light of vibrant health and peaceful living. She presents a workable scenario for living the integrated life of spirit, mind, and body. A modern Renaissance woman, Susan is a living example of the ancient wisdom, contemporary science, and twenty-first century vision that she teaches. Her workshops and books are powerful and life-transforming, and this CD interview touches on all of Susan's core teachings and explores the many facets that comprise living our best lives.

If you would like to learn more about Susan—how she got started in holistic health, her passions, and her secrets to healing your body, looking younger, and bringing your highest vision to fruition—then this is the perfect audio program for you. Susan is interviewed by radio personality Nick Lawrence, and together, they will uplift, inspire, motivate and empower you to create your best life. Their engaging, conversational interview brings Susan's message to vibrant life and holds your attention from beginning to end.

If you feel stuck in your life or like you're in a "spin-cycle" lifestyle...if you've lost some of your joy in living or you just need some gentle, loving, efficacious guidance to live in a more meaningful way...then *EveryDay Health—Pure & Simple* is perfect for you.

In this audio program, you will learn how to:

- Identify when stress is getting the best of you
- Deal with daily stresses with ease and grace
- Balance and integrate body, mind, and spirit
- Choose the best foods to heal your body
- Look younger with meditation, sleep, and raw foods
- Create healthy meals and snacks in only a few minutes
- Supercharge your energy and increase your endurance
- Protect yourself from obesity, diabetes, heart disease, and many cancers
- Raise healthy children with high self-esteem
- Stay motivated to exercise and accelerate fat loss
- Release bad habits easily and effortlessly
- Use gratitude to transform your life and create miracles
- Understand the healing power of solitude, silence, and Nature

- Become fearless and enthusiastic about your life
- Build your goal-seeking muscles and live your dreams
- Find your purpose and passion
- Use humor and laughter to awaken your highest potential
- Reignite self-esteem and strengthen your intuition
- Connect with your angelic helpers and Higher Power
- Make balance, peace, and joy your constant companions
- And so much more!

To order, please visit:

www.SusanSmithJones.com

A Fresh Start: Rejuvenate Your Life, Celebrate Life!, Choose to Live a Balanced Life, Make Your Life a Great Adventure, and more are available exclusively at: **www.SusansHealthyLiving.com.**

WE HAVE A BODY AND WE TAKE CARE OF IT. *We exercise, feed and bathe it. We have a mind and most of us exercise that, too. We read, write and think. But we also are a soul and if we don't nourish the soul, we won't be vibrantly healthy or complete.*

— SUSAN SMITH JONES

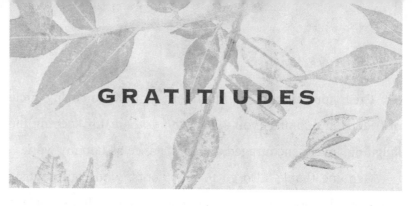

GRATITIUDES

If the only prayer you ever say in your life is "Thank you," this would suffice.
— MEISTER ECKHART

As I strive to live my dream with as much heart and grace as possible, I am blessed to have the encouragement of many people. It is my honor to express my appreciation to some special earth angels who played a vital role along the way.

First and foremost, my deepest gratitude goes to Gary Peattie and his superlative team at DeVorss & Co. What a blessing for me to work with such a committed, skillful group of people who embraced this project with enthusiasm. Thank you, Gary, for shepherding this book into existence, and for believing in me, advising me so wisely every step of the way, and for inspiring my best work.

My heartfelt gratitude goes to my editor, Catherine Viel, and her team at WriteCat Communications—Mary Lou Viel, Leo, and Ivan. Catherine's encouragement, patience, and expertise helped bring more life to my words in a nonintrusive, gentle way. You are a joy to work with and I appreciate our friendship.

Great appreciation and much love go to my amazing circle of friends and family (you know who you are)for keeping me laughing, loved, encouraged, and in balance as I do my work.

Genuine thanks also go to my clients, who continuously grant me the privilege of working with them. Thank you for letting me into your lives, and for trusting me to share your dreams, struggles, and successes in my books and during my radio and TV interviews.

For touching my heart in a special way with your wonderful music, thank you Steve Tyrell. During many of my writing days, your music fills my home and my heart with joy, inspiration, and passion.

I also want to thank all of the event coordinators for my keynote addresses, seminars, and workshops—for conferences, churches, businesses and companies, symposiums, and expos—who invite me to give motivational talks about holistic health and simple ways to create peaceful, balanced lives. It is a joy for me to have so many opportunities to speak with people worldwide and to spread the good news about living healthfully.

And heartfelt thanks to God, Christ, and the angels who nurture my spiritual side, enrich my life, and guide me along this magnificent journey with a gentle touch, wise counsel, and loving presence. Thank you for being the wind beneath my wings and showing me that with enough love, faith, trust, and patience, all challenges can be overcome and our dreams can become reality.

AT TIMES OUR OWN LIGHT GOES OUT *and is rekindled by a spark from another person. Think of those, with deep gratitude, who have lighted the flame within us.*

— ALBERT SCHWEITZER

ABOUT THE INCLUDED CD

Tucked into the back of this book you'll find a 77-minute audio CD which contains a heartening and uplifting interview with Susan that provides additional tips and tools you'll need to create an abundantly healthy, balanced life. It touches on all of Susan's core teachings and explores the many facets that comprise living our best lives. If you want to learn more about Susan—how she got started in holistic health, her passions, and her secrets to healing your body, looking younger, and bringing your highest vision to fruition—this is the perfect audio program for you and to share with your family and friends.

Susan is interviewed by radio personality Nick Lawrence, and together, they will inspire and empower you to create your best life. Their engaging, conversational interview brings Susan's message to vibrant life and will hold your attention from beginning to end. In her easygoing and motivational way, Susan will teach you how to: deal with daily stresses with ease and grace; choose the best foods to look and feel your best; accelerate fat loss; disease-proof your body; release bad habits; heal through silence and time in nature; reignite self-esteem; bring a sacred balance back into your life; and so much more!

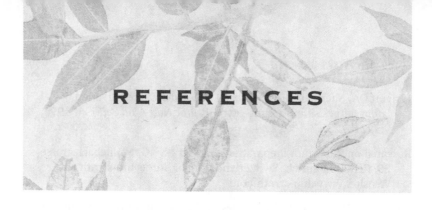

REFERENCES

Blumenthal J, Jiang W, et al. Stress management and exercise training in cardiac patients with myocardial ischemia; effects on prognosis and evaluation mechanisms. *Arch Int Med* 1997, Oct 27; 157:2213–2223.

Castillo-Richmond A, Schneider RH, et al. Effects of stress reduction on carotid artery atherosclerosis in hypertensive African Americans. *Stroke* 2000; 31:568–573.

Cohen S, Doyle WJ, Skoner DP, et al. Social ties and susceptibility to the common cold. *JAMA* 2004 Feb 15; 277(24):1940.

Glaser R, Kiecolt-Glaser JK. Stress-associated immune modulation and its implication for reactivation of latent herpes virus. In: Glaser R, Jones J eds. *Human Herpes Virus Infections*, New York, NY: Marcel Dekker Inc.; 1944:245–270.

Iso H, et al. Effects of mental stress on heart disease risk in Japanese men and women. *Circulation* 2002. August 13:106.

Kiecolt-Glaser JK, Marucha PT, et al. Slowing of wound healing by psychological stress. *Lancet* 1995;346:1194–1196.

Kuller LK. Dietary fat and chronic disease: epidemiologic overview. *J Am Diet Assoc* 1997; 97(7 Suppl):1906–1916.

LaVecchia C. Cancer associated with high-fat diets. *J Natl Cancer Inst Monogr* 1992; 12:79–85.

Macleod J, Smith GD, et al. Psychological stress and cardiovascular disease: empirical demonstration of bias in the prospective observational study of Scottish men. *Brit Med J* 2002 May 25; 324:1247 (abs).

Noll, George, et al. Mental stress induces prolonged endothelial dysfunction via endothelin-A receptors, rapid access issue; *Circulation* May 20, 2002.

Padgett DA, Sheridan JF, et al. Social stress and the reactivation of latent herpes simplex virus—type 1. *Proc Natl Acad Sci USA.* 1998; 9:7231–7235.

Research on Bio-Strath Preparations, Bio-Strath AG, Mühlebachstrasse 25, CH-8032 Zurich, Switzerland. E-mail: **info@bio-strath.ch**. Website: **www.bio-strath.com**

Steinmetz KA, Potter JD. Vegetables, fruit, and cancer prevention: a review. *J Am Diet Assoc.* 1996; 96(10):1027–1039.

Tavani A, La Vecchia C, Gallus S, et al. Red meat and cancer risk: a study in Italy. *Int J Cancer* 2000; 86(3):425–428.

> THE MOST INTELLIGENT WAY *to move in the direction of a good life is to live each day, each experience, as authentically as we can, with integrity, honesty, and courage."*
>
> – *Alexandra Stoddard*

BOOKS, MAGAZINES, RESOURCES & WEBSITES

Taking action galvanizes the spirit. When you do one thing,
you cut through that "stuck" feeling and build a momentum.

— ALEXANDRA STODDARD

Activated Air by Eng3. **www.eng3corp.com.**

Alt, Carol. *The RAW 50.* New York: Clarkson Potter/Publishers, 2007.

Barnard, Neal, M.D.. *Dr. Neal Barnard's Program for Reversing Diabetes.* Emmaus: Rodale, Inc., 2007.

Baroody, Theodore A., Ph.D., N.D., D.C. *Alkalize or Die.* Waynesville: Holographic Health Press, 8th Printing, 2002.

Brownstein, David, M.D. *Salt Your Way To Health.* West Bloomfield: Medical Alternatives Press, 2006.

Campbell, T. Colin, Ph.D. with Campbell, Thomas, M. II. *The China Study: Startling Implications for Diet, Weight Loss, and Long-Term Health.* Dallas: Benbella Books, 2005.

Cousens, Gabriel, M.D. *Conscious Eating.* Berkeley: North Atlantic Publishing, 2004.

Dement, William C., M.D. *The Promise of Sleep.* New York: Delacorte, 1999.

Dyer, Wayne W., Ph.D. *Change Your Thoughts—Change Your Life.* Carlsbad: Hay House, 2007.

Fife, Bruce, C.N., N.D. *The Coconut Oil Miracle.* New York: Avery, 2004.

Frawley, David Dr. Neti: *Healing Secrets of Yoga and Ayurveda.* Twin Lakes: Lotus Press, 2005.

Friends of Peace Pilgrim. **www.peacepilgrim.net.**

Fuhrman, Joel, M.D. *Cholesterol Protection for Life.* New Jersey: Gift of Health Press, 2006.

Gianni, Kevin, with Colameo, Annmarie. *The Busy Person's Fitness Solution.* Connecticut: A Better Life Press, 2007.

Good Medicine. **www.PCRM.org.**

Hallelujah Acres Diet & Lifestyle. **www.hacres.com.**

Hay, Louise. *Heal Your Body.* Carlsbad: Hay House, 2001.

Hay, Louise L., et al. *You Can Heal Your Life.* Directed by Michael Goorjian. Published by Hay House. Music by Jim Brickman. DVD movie. **1-800-654-5126.** 2007.

Health Science. **www.healthscience.org.**

Heber, David, M.D., Ph.D. *What Color is Your Diet?* New York: Regan Books, 2001.

Hintz, Rebecca Linder. *Healing Your Family History.* Carlsbad: Hay House, 2006.

Hocking, Melissa. *A Healing Initiation: Recognise the Healer Within.* Melbourne. Brolga Publishing, 2006.

Holick, Michael F., Ph.D., M.D. and Jenkins, Mark. *The UV Advantage.* New York: ibooks, 2003.

Jensen, Bernard, Dr. *Tissue Cleansing Through Bowel Management.* San Marcos: Bernard Jensen International, 2007.

Jones, Susan Smith. *Choose to Live Fully.* Camarillo: DeVorss & Co., 2009.

_____. *EveryDay Health—Pure & Simple.* Audio Program. Also available through **SusansHealthyLiving.com.**

_____. *Health Bliss: 50 Revitalizing NatureFoods & Lifestyle Choices to Promote Vibrant Health.* Carlsbad: Hay House, 2008.

_____. *Recipes for Health Bliss: Using NatureFoods to Rejuvenate Your Body & Life.* Carlsbad: Hay House, 2009.

_____. *Simplify • Detoxify • Meditate: Secrets to Making an Ordinary Life Extraordinary.* Carlsbad: Hay House, 2009. Also available through **SusansHealthyLiving.com.**

_____. *The Healing Power of NatureFoods: 50 Revitalizing SuperFoods & Lifestyle Choices to Promote Vibrant Health.* Carlsbad: Hay House, 2007.

_____ , and Warren, Dianne. *Vegetable Soup & The Fruit Bowl.* Sarasota: Oasis Publishing, 2007. To order, please call: **1-800-843-5743** (PT, M-F, 9-4).

_____. *Wired to Meditate, Celebrate Life!, Choose to Live Peacefully,* and many more Audio Programs. **www.SusanSmithJones.com**, **SusansHealthyLiving.com.**

Lindbergh, Anne Morrow. *Gift from the Sea.* New York: Pantheon Books, 1975.

Lisle, Douglas J., Ph.D., and Goldhamer, Alan, D.C. *The Pleasure Trap.* Summertown: Healthy Living Publications, 2003.

Vibrance. **www.livingnutrition.com.**

Malkmus, George H. *God's Way to Ultimate Health.* Shelby: Hallelujah Acres Publishing, 20th Printing, 2004.

Mars, Brigitte. *Rawsome!* North Bergen: Basic Health Publications, 2004.

Meyerwitz, Steve. *Water The Ultimate Cure.* Summertown: Book Publishing Company, 2001.

Moran, Victoria. *Fat, Broke & Lonely No More: Your Personal Solution to Overeating, Overspending, and Looking for Love in All the Wrong Places.* San Francisco: HarperOne, 2007.

Morin, Flechelle. *Kissing or No Kissing: Whom will You Save Your Kisses For.* San Diego: Cheval Publishing, 2006.

Neti Nasal Cleansing Pot. **www.ancient-secrets.com/neti.cfm.**

Nelson, Miriam, Ph.D. *Strong Women Stay Young.* New York: Bantam Books, 2000.

North American Vegetarian Scoiety. **www.vegetariansummerfest.org.**

Nungesser, Charles, Caralanne, and George. *How We All Went Raw.* Mesa: In the Beginning Health Ministry, 2007.

Nutrition Action Health Letter. **www.cspinet.org.**

Ornish, Dean, M.D. *The Spectrum.* New York: Random House, 2007.

Peeke, Pamela, M.D. *Fight Fat After Forty.* New York: Viking, 2000.

PhenomeNEWS. **www.phenomenews.com.**

Rhio. *Hooked on Raw: Rejuvenate Your Body and Soul with Nature's Living Foods.* New York: Beso Entertainment, 2000.

Romer, Leslie Van, DC. *Getting Into Your Pants.* Charlston: Advantage, 2008.

Ruiz, Don Miguel. *The Four Agreements.* San Rafael: Amber-Allen Publishing, 2000.

Sapolsky, Robert. *Why Zebras Don't Get Ulcers.* New York: W.H. Freeman & Company, 1999.

Seidman, Michael D. M.D. and Moneysmith, Marie. *Save Your Healing Now.* New York: Warner Wellness, 2006.

Smith, Lendon, M.D. *Happiness is a Healthy Life.* New York: McGraw-Hill, 1999.

Soria, Cherie. *Angel Foods.* Fort Bragg: The Book Publishing Company, 2003.

Stoddard, Alexandra. *Happiness for Two.* New York: Collins, 2008.

_____. *You Are Your Choices.* New York: Collins, 2007.

Tart-Jensen, Ellen. *Health is Your Birthright.* Berkeley: Celestial Arts, 2006.

The American Vegan Society. **www.americanvegan.org**

White Eagle. *The Quiet Mind.* Hampshire, England: The White Eagle Publishing Trust, 1972.

Women's Healing Org. International.

Wooden, John. *They Call Me Coach.* New York: McGraw-Hill, 2003.

Yogananda, Paramahansa. *Living Fearlessly.* Los Angeles: Self-Realization Fellowship Publications, 2003.

Your Body's Best Friend—MaxGXL Glutathione Supplement. **www.maxgxl.com/4healthyliving.** Click on *Preferred Customer.*

ABOUT THE AUTHOR

For a woman with three of America's most ordinary names, Susan Smith Jones, Ph.D., has certainly made extraordinary contributions in the fields of optimum health and fitness, anti-aging, nutritional medicine, alternative healthcare, and human potential. Selected as one of ten "Healthy American Fitness Leaders" by the President's Council on Physical Fitness and Sports, Susan is an award-winning writer and advice columnist.* She has authored 17 books and audio programs (including *Choose to Live Peacefully, Wired to Meditate, Vegetable Soup/The Fruit Bowl, The Healing Power of NatureFoods, Choose to Live Fully, Health Bliss, EveryDay Health—Pure & Simple, and Recipes for Health Bliss: Using NatureFoods to Rejuvenate Your Body & Life*) and hundreds of magazine articles, and she appears regularly on the covers of national and international publications. For thirty years, Susan taught students, staff, and faculty at UCLA how to be healthy and fit; she is a frequent guest on radio and television talk shows around the country. Topics she often discusses include simple ways to: look younger and live longer, boost immunity and energy, minimize stress and maximize joy, prevent and alleviate disease, use food as medicine, set up a healthful kitchen, create

---

* Other winners include Lance Armstrong, the late Ronald Reagan, former UCLA Basketball Coach John Wooden, Kathy Smith, Denise Austin, and Richard Simmons.

meals that rejuvenate the body, detoxify the body with whole foods and fresh juices, make healthful blender meals in seconds, raise healthy children, and bring a sacred balance into your body and life.

Susan is an acclaimed holistic lifestyle coach and private natural-foods chef who works with discerning clients around the world. She creates menus and rejuvenation programs designed to support and complement the needs of her individual clients, as well as the participants at her specialized holistic health retreats. In addition, she serves as a recipe developer and new-product consultant for the health industry.

Susan's inspiring message and innovative techniques for achieving total health in body, mind, and spirit have won her a grateful and enthusiastic following and have put her in constant demand internationally as a health and fitness consultant and motivational speaker (lectures, workshops, and keynote presentations) for community, corporate, and church groups. She is also founder and president of Health Unlimited, a Los Angeles–based consulting firm dedicated to the advancement of peaceful, balanced living and health education. A gifted teacher, Susan brings together modern research and ageless wisdom in all her work.

Many years ago, when a devastating car accident fractured Susan's back so badly that doctors told her she would never again be physically active and would live a life of chronic pain, she proved her doctors wrong. Her miraculous recovery proved to her that we all have within ourselves everything we need to live our lives to the fullest. She now regularly participates in a variety of fitness activities, including hiking, weight training, in-line skating, biking, Pilates™, horseback riding, and yoga. While she feels at home wherever she goes, Susan resides in West Los Angeles.

To order Susan's books, audiobooks, and other audio programs, visit:

www.SusanSmithJones.com,

www.SusansHealthyLiving.com,

or **www.PagingSusan.com**,

or call: **1-800-843-5743**.

To schedule a speaking engagement with Susan, please send complete details in writing at least four months in advance to:

Health Unlimited

P.O. Box 49215

Los Angeles, CA 90049

Attn. Manager

To order extra AUTOGRAPHED copies of this book (10 or more per order) to have on hand to give as gifts for birthdays, anniversaries, holidays, or any occasion, or to schedule a media interview with Susan, please call: **1-800-843-5743**.

"The doctor of the future will give no medicine, but will interest his patients in the care of the human frame, in diet, and in the cause and prevention of disease."

— THOMAS A. EDISON

"Cherish the music that stirs in your heart, the beauty that forms in your mind, the loveliness that drapes in your purest thoughts, for out of them will grow all delightful conditions, all heavenly environments; of these, if you but remain true to them, your world will at last be built."

— JAMES ALLEN

"We need to find God, and He cannot be found in noise and restlessness. God is the friend of silence."

— MOTHER TERESA

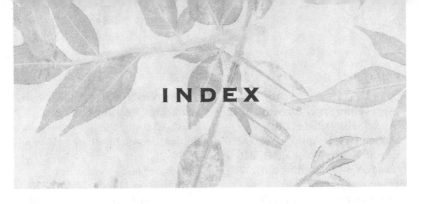

INDEX

G